No Gym Needed

Quick & Simple Workouts
for Gals on the Go
Get a Toned Body in
30 Minutes or Less!

Lise Cartwright

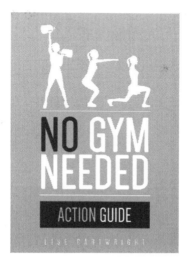

READ THIS FIRST

I've found that readers get the most success with this book when they use the Action Guide as they read along and do the workouts.

And just to say thanks for downloading my book, I'd love to give you access to some very special Video Lessons and the Action Guide for 100% FREE!

Visit http://lisecartwright.com/ngn-guide-access/ to Download

Dedication

Guy Cartwright, love of my life...

For always supporting me and pushing me to achieve my goals. Your love and encouraging words propelled me forward and your advice on healthy eating and exercise were a large driver behind allowing me to gain the knowledge and insight to write this book. Thank you xoxo

Table of Contents

INTRODUCTION

The Challenge

Breaking Down the Barriers to Staying Fit and Healthy

When's the last time you went to the gym or exercised? And when's the last time you actually enjoyed exercise or had the time to fit it into your hectic schedule?

Excuses, schedules and life in general can prevent you from staying fit and healthy. They stop you from losing weight, they stop you from maintaining your ideal weight and they stop you from fitting in time to exercise or change your lifestyle. Is it any wonder you're not feeling 100% happy with your weight and your body?

Picture this:

It's the beginning of the week, you've got your schedule all sorted and have set time aside to work out 3-4 times during that week. You're not a morning person, so after a normal workday is the best time to do your exercise, but when you get home from work late three days in a row, you're in no mood to exercise. Who wants to head to the gym and deal with all the gym bunnies and body-obsessed jocks when all you really want to do is take a shower, watch the latest episode of your favourite show and eat some yummy comfort food?

Does this scenario sound familiar to you?

Or maybe, this is more you:

You work from home and think you're pretty set when it comes to work/life balance. You work when you want to and meet with friends for lunch or take trips away when you want. You aim to exercise 4 times per week, and prefer to get it out of the way in the mornings. Yet you find yourself still sitting at your desk come 12pm, wondering where the morning went. By this time, the rest of your day is planned out and exercise is the last thing on your mind. Do this 2 or 3 days in a row and another week has gone by where your exercise routine has fallen by the wayside...

Whatever your situation is, we're all guilty of pushing aside exercise and healthy eating for things we consider more important, like work, client meetings or watching TV. We tell ourselves that tomorrow we'll start our exercise program or healthy lifestyle... **only to repeat the same actions week in and week out.**

With all of these barriers stopping us from getting fit, it's easy to see why exercise and staying healthy is one of the most popular categories in bookstores today. Yet there has never been (nor will there ever be) a book or program that answers every problem for every person.

But there is a book that provides solutions to your consistent exercise problems in ways that are easy to implement immediately into your life right now.

No Gym Needed: Quick & Simple Workouts for Gals on the Go has been developed to help you achieve a healthier lifestyle, allowing you to fit in exercises and routines that provide you with the results you want, in a succinct and easy-to-read manner. This book is for women who suffer from procrastination, lack of time, and a profane loathing for the gym and exercise in general.

As a full-time freelancer, entrepreneur, and previous 9-5er, I've mastered the art of choosing to fit exercise into my days and look after myself, without owning a gym membership or any special types of equipment. I've read and tested hundreds of different weight loss workouts and healthy lifestyle options to achieve a body and lifestyle I'm happy with.

Since I know you lack time (and perhaps the inclination) to do all of this research and testing, I've compiled the best weight loss and ideal weight maintenance workouts and created unique weekly and monthly programs for you. You'll find them all here in this book, ready to help you achieve a fit and healthy body.

Entrepreneurs, freelancers, office workers, students,

parents and many others who struggle with fitting in exercise and a healthy lifestyle, have already experienced success by implementing and taking action from the information provided in this helpful how-to guide.

Keri, a full-time, crazy-busy real estate agent from New Zealand, says, "The best thing about this book is you can jump straight to the section you need, find a routine or program and implement it within 30 minutes or less".

Lizzie, a full-time freelancer and sometime traveller from New York, uses the book to help maintain her weight. Lizzie believes the biggest benefit of *No Gym Needed* is that it "gives you the steps to take to implement exercise into your schedule with no fluff and no BS, allowing you to jump straight into the heart of it all - working out".

Although this book is designed to help you lose weight and adopt a healthier lifestyle, those goals still require effort on your part. If you don't actually do the exercises, nothing will change. It's as simple as that.

Even if you've been exercising for a while or trying to lose weight, this book will still hit home for you in a way that other programs have not. Here's what Florence, a full-time traveller and entrepreneur from Ireland, had to say:

"As someone who is constantly battling with weight, travelling and maintaining a freelance business, I know that without *No Gym Needed*, I wouldn't have been able to implement exercise into my schedule. This book will work for anyone and everyone".

The ideas, routines and workouts presented in this book can be implemented and actioned by anyone, anywhere, and they will instantly provide you with ways to start exercising and feeling healthy today. Whether you're stuck working in an office, working from home, juggling multiple start-ups, jobs, or chasing the kids around the house, there is a routine in here that will work for you.

As you read on, you'll learn how I went from struggling to get 1-2 days a week of exercise in and 22 pounds (10 kg) overweight, to reaching my ideal weight, exercising 5 times per week without setting foot anywhere near a gym or exercising for longer than 30 minutes at a time.

I've spent the last 2 years working full-time as a freelancer, and during this time, I have tested hundreds of ideas, tips, hacks and routines around weight loss and maintaining weight loss. This has allowed me to learn, through trial and error, about ways I can maintain a healthy lifestyle without having to join a gym or spend hours exercising for little to no change.

Throughout this book, you'll come across the following:

- **Total Body Workouts** to try so that you can work out the routines that best fit your lifestyle and keep you interested
- **30-Day Programs** to help you kick-start your exercising and develop a habit
- **Lifestyle Hacks** (or clever solutions) that will instantly provide you with ways to stay fit and healthy, no matter what you do on a day-to-day basis

In the words of Aristotle, "We are what we repeatedly do".

No Gym Needed provides you with clear and actionable steps to get the body you want. It is straight to the point and will help you achieve your fitness goals, while taking 30 minutes (or less!) of your day.

I promise that if you follow the how-to's and hacks and routines, you'll achieve your weight loss and fitness goals 3X faster than what you're currently doing. AND I promise that you'll achieve a more balanced work/life day, where you can spend time with friends and family, and also achieve your work goals while meeting your exercise needs.

Not only that, but if you stick to the ideas and routines laid out in the book and complete the 14-Day Challenge (available in the free Action Guide) at the end, you'll create new habits and see a change in how you approach your day, leading to a healthier lifestyle and a hot, toned body to boot. Win-win, right?

Before you jump straight in, I'd like to share something with you that should be kept in mind while reading the book. By following this one piece of advice, you put yourself in the top 10% of successful people. **People who follow this advice successfully achieve their weight loss and lifestyle goals faster, while 90% of unsuccessful people choose to ignore it.**

Failure to follow this one idea leads to unhealthy lifestyle habits and weight gain, rather than weight loss.

Are you ready for it? Here it is...

Learn, Then Do.

If you want to be successful at anything in life, you have to take action. But where successful people excel over unsuccessful people is that they understand the art of learning then doing, and applying this learning quickly.

People who lose weight and maintain their weight loss do so because of consistent habits. They learn quickly and then implement what works immediately. How many times have you looked at yourself in the mirror and wished you could be thinner, healthier, more toned – but never took the steps to do something about it?

Don't be the person who wishes they could change the

way they look, but doesn't do anything to make the necessary changes. Be the kind of person that other people want to be. Be the kind of person other people see and say, "I don't know how they fit in the time to LOOK THAT GOOD!" Be the kind of person who implements what they learn, who takes action and does so quickly.

The only people who shouldn't continue reading this book are those that have the body and lifestyle they want. For the rest of us, there's always room to grow and change and if you're not happy with your body or lifestyle, then this book is just for you.

The ideas, routines and lifestyle hacks you're about to read have been **proven to create body-changing and long-lasting results**. All you have to do to achieve the body you want is to keep reading.

Each chapter will provide insights as you strive to fit exercise into your life and achieve your weight-loss goals.

Take control of your time right now. Make it work for you and create a body you love.

CHAPTER 1 - WHY THIS BOOK?

How It All Started...

After 18 months working from home, self-employed, I had gained extra weight, felt really lethargic and was not 100% happy with the way I looked. In short, I had an honest distaste for my body. Don't get me wrong; I LOVED working for myself and being at home, surrounded by all my creature comforts, never having to get dressed up or leave the house if I didn't want to. And here lay part of the problem for me.

It got to a point where I loathed having to dress up to go out of the house. Mainly because nothing fit anymore, jeans were tight, tops were less than figure enhancing. Coupled with not having exercised for at least 6 months, I was feeling like a big heifer (translation - big moo cow!), with no reason to really venture out anywhere.

Something had to change.

So I did what any sane person would do - I Googled it, of course! Isn't that the answer for everything we don't know these days? It's certainly my go-to reaction for everything I don't know the answer to.

What did I Google? "How to lose weight WITHOUT going

to the gym Because if there's one thing I hate with pure loathing, it's going to the gym. Whether it's a male/female or all-female gym, there's just no way that I can step foot in one of those institutions. Why? Let me tell you...

Picture this:

You're carrying a few extra pounds here and there, things are a little jiggly but hey, your clothes still fit (albeit with a few muffin tops and bulges appearing here and there). You decide it's time to start exercising again because summer is around the corner and you love to hit the beach. In your current form, donning a bikini or any form of bathing suit sends you into a state of mass terror.

So, you make an appointment to visit your local gym. And yes, you have to make an appointment because they are so busy; you can no longer just drop in. Plus, they want time to prepare and figure out how they can hook you into as many things as possible... You go to the gym, meet with a body-obsessed male who is also a personal trainer and he goes over the facilities, the benefits of classes and how this gym provides one-on-one personal training for those who need it. He then follows up with, "So when can I book your first personal training session?"

Did I also mention I'm not a fan of personal trainers?

Now, you're all signed up and ready to hit the gym. You

look at your schedule... the gym is about a 10-minute drive from you, so it's going to take some effort to get there in the early morning, which is when you think it will fit in best with your daily routine. So you set your alarm for 6am the next morning. Alarm goes off, you hit snooze twice and jump out of bed at 6.30am. You suddenly remember you're meant to be hitting the gym. Um, that's not going to work now. You've got a client call at 7.30am and then some work that is due by 11am, so going to the gym now just isn't going to work. You reschedule it for 3.30pm.

3.30pm - Crap, you're still in the middle of writing a witty Facebook retort to a friend's post, so you push the gym till later, aiming for 5pm. 5pm arrives, you chuck some gear on and head to the gym, where you're met with 50 other people all vying for the same exercise equipment. You check the class schedule and see that there is a body pump class in 10 minutes so you decide to join that instead of waiting for equipment to be free. You join the class and proceed to drop your weights several times, whack someone on the bum with your bar, and let a fart or two slip out while you're doing the clean and press...

This. Was. Me. Stop laughing!

I could continue on with other experiences, but I'm sure you get the gist. Fitting in exercise and going to the gym just didn't gel well with my current lifestyle or me.

So getting back to my Google search... I found a LOT of options, but figuring out what would get me the greatest amount of weight loss in the least amount of time, wasn't immediately clear. I was looking for routines I could do in 30 minutes or less, but would also provide me with maximum weight loss.

Confusion ensued. Who could I trust? It doesn't take a brainiac to figure out that anyone can put up exercise routines touting that they will help you lose weight and get fit. I was flooded with thoughts like, "Is this routine safe?", "Do I need weights?", and "Am I doing this right?" – all valid questions.

Through trial and error (and a little pain), I figured out the routines that worked and got rid of the ones that didn't (leaving some scathing comments on blogs in the process!). By reading this book, you can avoid all of this confusion and know that EVERY routine has been human-tested by me. No animals were harmed in the writing of this book!

The ideas and hacks that you'll be presented with throughout the book are all personally tested and tried by me. Everything you read in here has worked for me. Using the routines and hacks in this book, I've created a lifestyle that I now enjoy and have a body I'm beginning to enjoy again, as is my husband...

The book is split up into three sections:

1. Section 1: Chapters 1-3 cover the basic concepts and introduction to the book,
2. Section 2: Chapters 4-6 focus on specific weight loss and ideal weight maintenance routines as well as best practices around form, and
3. Section 3: Chapters 7-9 focus on the 14-Day Challenge and other important details to help continue on your path to a body you'll love.

Section 2 is where you'll find specific routines targeting weight loss, with body-weight and weighted exercise options (use household items only!), as well as routines to help you maintain your ideal weight.

I wanted to provide routines for weight loss and weight management because the routines and frequency of executing them are different depending on what your goals are.

In the next chapter, I'm going to go over the solution I've developed to solve the issue of fitting exercise into your life without needing to join a gym. We'll discuss some lifestyle hacks here as well. Read on to better understand the solutions and learn how you should get started.

CHAPTER 2 - THE SOLUTION

What I Discovered

As I researched and tried different routines and ideas, I started seeing that there were some core exercises that could be used to design the body I wanted. There were also some lifestyle hacks I could apply to my day, so that I could actually fit in exercise. Part of this process included discovering that I didn't need to belong to a gym, nor did I need to exercise for hours at a time to achieve the results I wanted - a toned body that I WAS HAPPY with.

That last little sentence is really important. Before you begin any form of exercising, you need to determine why or who you're doing this for. You need to realise that you should only be doing this for yourself.

I'm curvy, and I'm always going to be that way, so my goal was to tone and firm. I wanted to work *with* my curves rather than against them. I feel that this is one area that most people struggle with, particularly if you're like me and read magazines. How many magazines do you see that show curvy women? All I ever see are perfect bodies and tight abs, butts and thighs.

Those women have been airbrushed to within a breath

of their "normal" body. How can anyone ever hope to look like that without making significant lifestyle changes and spending some serious moola?

This is exactly my point! You can't (or maybe you're lucky and can - awesome for you!). Your best option is to work with the body shape you have and tone it so that it looks its best. We are not all the same, so not only will you find weight loss and weight maintenance routines in this book, but you'll find routines for specific areas of your body, so you can target the areas that you feel need work the most.

You'll also find routines that take less than 30 minutes to complete.

We all have the same amount of hours in a day. How we choose to spend them is entirely up to us. My philosophy has always been to work smarter, so I love hacks – tricks and clever solutions – that allow me to get the same result but in less time. This is what you'll find throughout this book - ideas, routines and hacks that provide you with exercise options that can slot into 30 minutes of time during your day.

What's Required From You

Along the way, you're going to need to decide if you actually want to be healthy and fit - which I'm assuming you do, otherwise why are you reading this book? Part of the process of fitting exercise into your day is about developing habits, and you'll get plenty of help and advice from this book about how to do this, and how to exercise quickly while still getting the results you're after.

To make life easier, make sure you visit the free fast-track page (details on how to access the page are in Chapter 4) so that you can access the routines, videos, hacks and apps without having to flick through the entire book to find them.

A large part of losing weight or designing the body you want relies on understanding the changes in your body. This is why we need to track and measure our progress. Don't worry; you don't have to weigh yourself if you don't want to. It's not necessary to track and measure your actual weight. Instead, we'll focus on taking more meaningful measurements, such as your upper-thigh measurement or your hip and waist measurements. What are we measuring? Body fat. This is a much better indicator of weight loss and body design than what the scales say.

If you didn't know already, muscle is much heavier than fat, so even if you have been working your butt off for a few weeks, the scales may not immediately reflect weight loss because you're building muscle. By measuring parts of your body, you can see where fat is being replaced with muscle. It's a far better motivator when you see centimetres (or inches) melting away than jumping on scales that tell you that you haven't lost any weight.

You'll be provided with different ways to track and measure your progress - but don't get too hung up on this area. There are lots of apps and programs you can use, but if you want to keep it simple, pen and paper works just as well. You'll have options, so choose what makes the most sense to you, but provides you with the quickest way to get started. For me, I choose pen and paper to begin with.

Lifestyle Hack

I found the act of physically writing it down makes it more real for me and creates the habit faster. You can learn more about this process by reading an article that details it over at www.lifehack.org/articles/ productivity/writing-and-remembering-why-we-remember-what-we-write.html.

A Word About Routines

As I've already mentioned, this book provides you with lifestyle hacks and ways to stay fit and healthy no matter what your schedule is like. But, you also get access to the routines I've used to lose weight and maintain my target weight.

As I've already discussed, the bulk of this book has been

split into two sections, one focused on weight loss and one focused on maintaining your ideal weight once you've reached it. Both sections include body-weight exercises and weighted exercises (using household items). So don't worry, you don't have to run out and buy any equipment.

If you do want to look at buying equipment, like dumbbells and kettle bells, these details are provided in the weighted sections.

And don't worry; all the weighted exercises are based on normal, everyday household items that you'll already likely have lying around the house.

What to Expect

This how-to guide is a full compilation of my successes, failures and wasted energy, simplified into 3 easy-to-follow sections.

By now you should have downloaded the Action Guide (http://lisecartwright.com/ngn-guide-access/) and learned that the fast-track page is where all the 'special sauce' stuff is at, but if you haven't, you will learn more in Chapter 4 and get the information you need to access the fast-track page.

The Action Guide and access to the the fast-track page is included with the purchase of your book, and you're going to want to access both to complete your body-shape identification (Chapter 4) and to track and measure your progress.

Are you ready to get started? In the next section, we're going to make sure that you've got the right form. Without correct form, you could damage yourself; target the wrong muscles and just look plain silly while doing a move. We'll also look at safety while you're exercising, as this is something else you need to factor into your exercise habits.

CHAPTER 3 - FORM & SAFETY

Body Awareness

Before you start any form of exercise, it's important that you think about the types of exercises you'll be doing and where you plan to do them.

If you don't have the correct form, you may not benefit from the exercise in the right way, because you're not targeting the right muscle, or you could end up damaging yourself instead.

If you're not aware of your surroundings, or don't let others know what your exercise plans are, you could find yourself in some icky situations.

Read on to avoid any negative outcomes that prevent you from achieving your exercise goals.

Form

Before you start working out, you need to make sure that you understand how to protect yourself from injuries. Learning the correct form for each exercise is important. If you don't learn how to do an exercise the right way, you could end up damaging your back or muscles, or you could end up targeting the wrong muscle group, which defeats the original purpose of the exercise.

No one wants to end up with a "stuffed" back because they didn't take the time to read and execute how to do a specific exercise. So, even if you've been exercising for a while, make sure you check your form by watching yourself in a mirror as you do each exercise or by following the steps below.

Each routine provides you with specific instructions on how to do each move, but if you want to make sure your form is correct (which you totally should), then this is what you need to know.

Upper and Lower Body Exercises

Follow these steps to ensure that you're protecting yourself from injury:

1. When using any type of weight, never jerk the weight behind you or above your head. You want to aim for a fluid, deliberate motion. Also, make sure that you've got a good grip on them, particularly if you're doing squats and have the weights resting on your thighs or shoulders. Make sure the weights are secure before you begin the exercise move.

2. When working on your back or core muscles, always make sure that your core is pulled tight. This means pulling your belly button into your back, basically sucking your tummy in. You need

to keep it that way the whole time you're working on your back or core area. This prevents lower back injury and pulled abdominal muscles.

3. Never fully extend your arms, and keep your elbows soft, particularly when you're using weights of any kind (household items included). If you fully extend and lock your elbows in place, you risk injuring your biceps, triceps and elbow joints. Also, when doing lunges or squats, never lock your knees in place as you're coming up; always keep them soft. This protects your knees and keeps the muscles you're targeting engaged and working.

4. When working on any part of your upper or lower body, keep your stance soft. This means keeping your knees slightly bent and your weight pushing through your heels, particularly when you're using weights. This will help keep you balanced and takes some of the pressure off your upper body.

Watch the video on the fast-track page to see all of these tips in action!(Log-in details in Chapter 4)

Exercise Hack

No matter what exercise you're doing, always suck your belly button into your lower back. This ensures that you're protecting your lower back at all times and helps prevent injuries developing.

Safety Best Practices

While the above is focused on form, this area is focused on making sure you're safe while you work out, particularly if you're working out alone or outdoors. This is where planning and scheduling your exercise is key. You need to think about where you're going to exercise ahead of time so that you can ensure your own safety.

Some things to consider as you're exercising:

1. If you're working out alone, make sure that someone knows what you're doing, particularly if you're using weights of any kind. This is especially true if you work from home and no one will be home to see you until after 5pm. The easiest way for me to do this is to check in with my husband at lunchtime. That way, if he doesn't hear from me, he knows something's up.

2. If you're planning to workout outside, let someone know where you'll be, particularly if you're going for a run and have your headphones in or you're working out at a park in the middle of the day. Make sure you are aware of your surroundings and of anyone else around you.

3. Be smart about the weights you're using, particularly if you opt to use dumbbells or kettle bells. Don't increase weight amounts too quickly, or you could end up causing yourself some

serious damage. Always start light and, if after 3 days it feels too easy, increase the weight until it's hard but not impossible.

There is no harm in being smart and being aware. If you work out by yourself, always let someone know what you're up to, even if it's a quick post on Facebook or tweet on Twitter. Heck, you could even take a pic and pop it on Instagram. Just leave out your actual location, of course.

Stretching

At the end of each routine you need to stretch, even if you've only got a couple of minutes. Believe me, I learned the hard way. You don't want your muscles to be screaming at you tomorrow morning and the next, and you won't be able to work out. Again, I learned the hard way...

I remember a program that I started a few years ago called the "butt, thigh and leg workout" that was all about targeting those 3 main areas using a weighted belt. The first few days were hard, but I loved the feeling of working out my butt and thighs - problem areas for me because I'm pear-shaped.

Anyway, on the third day, I literally could not walk. Picture this if you can (and I'm sure you will!):

At the time, I was living in a 2-story townhouse and my bedroom was upstairs. I went up to bed on day 2, and by day 3 I couldn't even walk, let alone face walking down a flight of stairs. What did I do instead? Yep, I had to sit down at the top and butt-scoot down a flight of 20 stairs (much to the delight of my roommates at the time). I don't know what was worse, the pain or the embarrassment!

Had I taken the time to stretch my muscles on days 1

and 2, I would have been sore on day 3, but it's unlikely a flight of stairs would have kicked my ass. Lesson learned.

So, if you want to avoid doing the "butt walk of shame", you need to make time to stretch.

In case you need more reasons, here are 5 benefits you'll get from stretching besides avoiding injury:

1. **Circulation**

    Your muscles work hard when you're working out, so hard that blood circulation can slow down, preventing nutrients reaching your muscles. This is a large part of why your muscles hurt the next day, and why you should stretch. By stretching, you increase blood flow and the nutrients can then be supplied to your muscles when they need them most. This reduces soreness and allows you to exercise those same muscles the following day.

2. **Flexibility**

    This is just common sense. The more flexible you are, the easier exercising becomes and the less strain there is on major areas of your body. As you get older, your muscles become shorter and tighter, so the more you stretch, the more you lengthen those muscles and the longer they'll be able to support you.

3. **Joint Motion**

By stretching, you increase your level of flexibility, which leads to an increase in motion for your joints. It's win-win as far as I can see. Range of motion becomes important the older you get, so do yourself a favour and stretch whenever you work out to ensure that you have the use of your muscles for many, many years to come.

4. **Stress Reduction**

Along with exercising, stretching also helps to reduce stress, not just on your mind, but also on your body. By stretching, you release the tension in your muscles, not just from working out, but also from the stress of the day. You'll also release endorphins, just like you do while exercising, which will help to improve your mood and the way you feel overall.

5. **Reduce Lower Back Pain**

Stretching also helps to relieve tension you have built up in your lower back during an exercise session. Chronic lower back pain is one of the most common ailments that people deal with, so stretching this area will help relieve the pain and help strengthen back muscles as well.

Now that you understand just how important it is, make sure you refer to the fast-track page for the list of the top 10 stretches you should do following each workout.

Now that we've covered form and stretching, you can dive into the meaty chapters and start exercising! Read on to learn how your body shape plays a part in the types of exercises you should do, and then determine which routines best suit your shape. Start your exercise regimen and journey to having an awesome body in 30 minutes or less - no gym needed!

CHAPTER 4 - WEIGHT LOSS

Body Shape

Weight loss and maintenance can be difficult, but only when you don't understand your body and what it needs to operate at its optimal level.

Let's start with looking at the different body shapes and identifying the one that most closely represents you.

Body Shapes

There are 4 main body shapes, as shown in the image below:

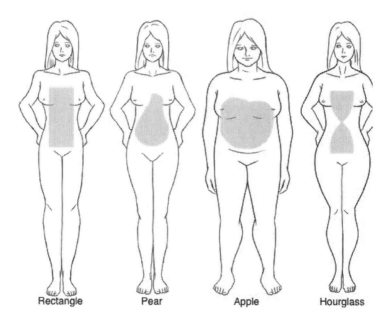

Rectangle   Pear   Apple   Hourglass

Let's break them down and look at them closer. Just in case you're not 100% sure what you are, the descriptions below will help.

Rectangle: you're this body shape if your shoulder and hip areas are the same size, your waist is slim and you're nice and tall with long legs. You probably have no problem finding clothes that fit, except for trousers, which can sometimes be too short.

Pear: you're this body shape if your hips are larger than your bust area and your waist slopes out to your hip area. Basically, you're smaller up top than you are around your hips and you tend to carry most of your weight in the hip area.

Apple: you're this body shape if your tummy area is larger than any other part of your body. You'll find that your shoulders are probably rounded and you tend to carry most of your weight around your waist and tummy area.

Hourglass: you're this body shape if your hips and bust areas are the same proportion and your waist is small. This shape gives you a lot of curves and is what some refer to as a "classic" woman's shape.

Using the fast-track page, make note of your body shape by circling the image in the workouts PDF. This way you've got a quick reference to refer back to when it comes time to exercise and determine which routines will work best for your shape.

Looking at the image above, determine your body shape and then move on to the next part of the chapter where you'll see the types of routines best suited for your shape.

Side Note: Don't forget to record this information so that you always have it as a reference. Your body shape will never change, unless you choose to surgically change it. Learn to work with it and you'll have a much easier time with losing and maintaining your weight.

Weight Loss

Welcome to the **Weight Loss** section. The routines, hacks and ideas presented here are all focused on losing weight.

As I've already highlighted, losing weight can be tough, but only when you don't know how your body works or what areas you should be targeting.

You should already know what your body shape is. If you don't, go back to the body shape identification area and figure this out. If you don't do this, you could find your weight loss slow and a little frustrating.

Beside each routine, there will be an indicator as to which body shape this routine targets. With the create-your-own-routine options (shown in Chapter 8), each exercise will also tell you which body shape the exercise is best suited for, as it targets a specific area for that body shape.

No matter what your body shape, you should always ensure that you are aiming for total body workouts. Use body-weight or weighted exercises to target your trouble areas, and use cardio (if you want fast weight loss) to get a full workout.

The routines in this chapter are split into two different sections:

1. Body-weight Routines
2. Weighted Routines (using household items)

The aim is to choose the exercises and routines that work best for your body shape. The body shape indicators, beside routines, will guide you so you'll immediately know which ones are just right for you.

Top 10 Diet Tips

- If you're planning to work out in the morning, eat a big breakfast. Aim for eggs, spinach and other vegetables for this meal. And don't think small here, go big. A big breakfast will actually reduce hunger and promote weight loss as it kicks your metabolism into gear. Just make sure it's full of good foods, not heavy carbs. Think slow-carb here.

- Can't stomach a big breakfast? Eat low fat/ high protein/moderate carb meals instead. Some examples are fruit smoothies with protein powder, raisins & protein powder, grilled chicken & fruit salad, oatmeal with cinnamon. You get the gist.

- Eat low carb/high protein/moderate fat meals only in the evening; avoid eating these at any other time of the day. These include things like soups, stir-frys, salads, crunchy veggies and red meat.

- For lunch, you can eat either low fat/high protein/moderate carb or low carb/high protein/moderate fat depending on when you're exercising. If no exercise in the afternoon, stick with low carb/high protein/ moderate fat, but if you are exercising in the afternoon, then you'll want to choose low fat/high protein/moderate carb so that you've got energy.

- Make sure you eat protein at every meal. This doesn't mean red meat or a chicken breast; it could simply mean adding a scope of protein powder to each meal - easy to do. This will reduce your appetite, reduce the afternoon "brain-fog" and if you are dieting will reduce muscle-mass loss.

- Don't drink your calories. Think about that every time you hit Starbucks or any cafe. If you're grabbing a coffee, do you need that cream on top? What about an iced coffee? Do you have cream on that too? Avoid drinking calories by avoiding these foods during the week. Have them on your cheat day instead.

- Give up bread. It's simple. You'll feel 100% better just by doing this one thing. Have you read the book "Wheat Belly"? It's an interesting read and one of the reasons why I have cut all bread out of my diet.

- Drink more water and white, green, oolong,

black or herbal tea. Reach for this instead of juice or soda. Leave these to your cheat day.

- Take an Omega 3 supplement every night before you go to bed. You need these to combat the high level of Omega 6 oils that are more common in our diet than they used to be. Take before bed and let them work their magic.

Always have healthy snacks available. In your bag, on your desk, in the car, around your house – just have them on hand. What's healthy? Protein powder or meal replacement powder + water, nuts and seeds, baby carrots, etc. Leave everything else until cheat day.

A Word on Regularity

When it comes to how often you should exercise when you're trying to lose weight, there are a couple of points to keep in mind:

- If you're training with any type of weights, you need to allow 24-48 hours of rest between weighted exercises to allow muscles to repair themselves. Keep this in mind when you're using any of the weighted exercise routines.
- The ideal weight loss regimen with weights is 2-3 times per week.
- With cardio exercises, you can do these more frequently, up to 3-5 times per week.

- For optimal weight loss, aim to exercise 5 times per week, bearing in mind weights and cardio best practices.
- If you want to lose weight fast, do cardio 5 times per week and add some of the weighted exercises to your routines 3 times per week.

Ready? Let's get started! Turn the page to learn about your first workout routine!

Body Weight Routines

If you're just starting out, body-weight routines are your best option. I started off here because I hadn't been exercising regularly for a good 4 months. You don't want to do any damage, so if you're unsure about what is best for you, seek the advice of your medical practitioner. I am by no means a doctor; I just worked my way through lots of different routines until I found the ones that worked best for me. Then, I asked friends with differing body shapes to test routines I'd identified as being best for their bodies. This chapter outlines the best options as tested by us.

Always start off light and don't push yourself too hard in the first few days. Once you've been exercising regularly, you can start to increase reps and really think about your form and how you can push yourself more.

Below you'll find a 14-day workout chart and a 30-day workout chart that you can use to lose weight. None of these routines require any weights, so they are ideal for beginners or if you're travelling.

Below this, you'll also find some go-to exercises, HIIT (High Intensity Interval Training) workouts and total-body workouts as well, just so you can mix things up. If you want to create your own routine, refer to the Chapter 8 for more details about how to best do this.

14-Day Workout - Kick-starting the Weight Loss

Use this if you haven't been exercising for a while and need to ease yourself back into exercising and setting up regular routines:

14-Day Program

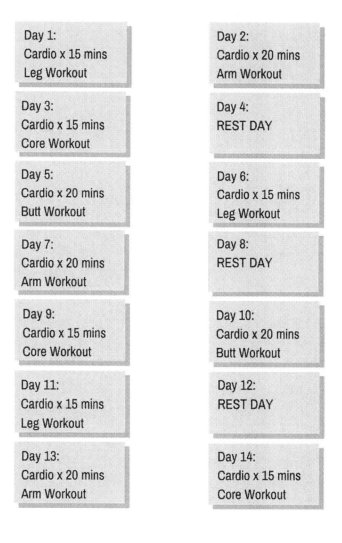

Day 1: Cardio x 15 mins Leg Workout	Day 2: Cardio x 20 mins Arm Workout
Day 3: Cardio x 15 mins Core Workout	Day 4: REST DAY
Day 5: Cardio x 20 mins Butt Workout	Day 6: Cardio x 15 mins Leg Workout
Day 7: Cardio x 20 mins Arm Workout	Day 8: REST DAY
Day 9: Cardio x 15 mins Core Workout	Day 10: Cardio x 20 mins Butt Workout
Day 11: Cardio x 15 mins Leg Workout	Day 12: REST DAY
Day 13: Cardio x 20 mins Arm Workout	Day 14: Cardio x 15 mins Core Workout

30-Day Workout - Continuing the Weight Loss

Use this chart if you've been exercising on and off but

haven't noticed any major weight loss. Continue with this routine for 3 months and you'll be able to decide whether you need to make any changes, such as increasing reps or adding weights, or whether you're ready to head to the next section, which is all about maintaining your ideal weight.

Day 1 Cardio x 20 min Butt Workout	Day 2 Cardio x 20 min Arm Workout	Day 3 Cardio x 20 min Core Workout
Day 4 REST DAY	Day 5 Cardio x 20 min Leg Workout	Day 6 Cardio x 20 min Butt Workout
Day 7 Cardio x 20 min Arm Workout	Day 8 REST DAY	Day 9 Cardio x 20 min Core Workout
Day 10 Cardio x 20 min Butt Workout	Day 11 Cardio x 20 min Arm Workout	Day 12 REST DAY
Day 13 Cardio x 20 min Leg Workout	Day 14 Cardio x 20 min Butt Workout	Day 15 Cardio x 20 min Arm Workout
Day 16 REST DAY	Day 17 Cardio x 20 min Core Workout	Day 18 Cardio x 20 min Butt Workout
Day 19 Cardio x 20 min Arm Workout	Day 20 REST DAY	Day 21 Cardio x 20 min Core Workout
Day 22 Cardio x 20 min Leg Workout	Day 23 Cardio x 20 min Butt Workout	Day 24 REST DAY
Day 25 Cardio x 20 min Arm Workout	Day 26 Cardio x 20 min Core Workout	Day 27 Cardio x 20 min Leg Workout
Day 28 REST DAY	Day 29 Cardio x 20 min Butt Workout	Day 30 Cardio x 20 min Arm Workout

30-Day Program

Cardio Options:

1. One-Room Cardio 15-Minute Workout (by
   backonpointe.tumblr.com) - start on the left-hand

side reading downwards:

One Room Cardio

20 jumping jacks	30 jumping jacks
:30 sec high knees	:40 sec jump rope
:30 sec butt kickers	5 burpees
5 jump squats	:20 sec jog in place
10 front kicks	:15 sec run in place
:30 sec mountain climbers	:30 sec water break
:30 sec water break	20 jumping jacks
5 burpees	10 lateral jumps
20 jumping jacks	5 jump squats
:30 sec jump rope	:30 sec jump rope
5 split jump squats	5 tuck jumps
10 front kicks	:30 sec water break
:30 sec march	20 jumping jacks
:15 sec high knees	:25 sec high knees
:15 sec butt kickers	5 squats
:30 sec water break	:40 sec march (finish)

2. 20-Minute High Intensity Workout (by backonpointe.tumblr.com) - repeat twice:

20 Min HITT

1 min jumping jacks
:30 sec side lunges
:30 sec squats
1 min jog in place
:30 sec burpees
:30 sec lunges
1 min jump rope
:30 sec mountain climbers
:30 speed skaters
1 min butt kickers
:30 sec lunge kicks
:30 sec squats
1 min march in place
:30 sec side lunges
:30 sec push-ups

Leg, Arm, Core & Butt Workout Options:

1. Leg Workouts

- 10 x high knees, 20 x deep squats & 25 x calf raises (increase by 5 reps each day) or
- 10 x butt kicks, 20 x calf raises & 25 x lunges each leg (increase by 5 reps each day)

2. Arm Workouts

- 10 x push-ups, 20 x seated dips & 25 x shoulder tap in plank (increase by 5 reps each day) or
- 10 x seated dips, 20 x wide arm push-ups & 25 x front punches each arm - alternate (increase by 5 reps each day)

3. Core Workouts

- 10 sec side plank (both sides), 20 Russian twists & 25 leg raises (increase by 5 reps each day) or
- 10 x side bends (each side), 20 x leg raises & 25 Russian twists (increase by 5 reps each day)

4. Butt Workouts

- 10 x burpees, 20 x lunges (each leg) & 25 squats (increase by 5 reps each day) or
- 10 x burpees, 20 x pile squats & 25 x walking lunges each leg (increase by 5 reps each day)

Refer to the fast-track page for videos on how to do these workouts plus all the other information you'll need throughout this book.

To access the fast-track page, visit this link: http:// lisecartwright.com/ngn-fast-track-page and use the following details to access:

Password: 6KAZKUfVAXT4

These are just for owners of the NGN book, so please don't share them with anyone else!

Exercise Hacks

Hack 1 - If you want to reduce your blood pressure and increase your deep sleep cycles, exercise in the morning, before 11am. A study conducted by Appalachian State University (www.news.appstate.edu/2011/06/13/ early-morning-exercise/) found that people who exercised in the mornings spent up to 75% more time in reparative "deep sleep" than those who exercised later in the day.

Hack 2 - Look at adding intermittent fasting to your diet (visit www.lifehack.org/articles/lifestyle/intermittent-fasting-the-ultimate-weight-loss-hack.html) . This post from Nerd Fitness goes into all the nerdy details.

Studies show that you can lose 2-3 pounds (0.9 - 1.3 kilograms) per week through fasting. Start with fasting for 12 hours each day and work your way up to 16-20 hours (with 20 hours being the maximum time to fast) per day. This is a great way to burn excess body fat quickly and safely. Make sure you check out this diet properly before starting it!

Hack 3 - Eat less than 75 grams of carbs per day while you're looking to lose weight. 75 grams is equal to 1.5 cups of rice, 2 slices of bread or 18 ounces of cola. Doing this one thing can help you to lose up to 3 pounds (1.3 kg) per week plus whatever you lose working out.

Turn the page to see how to incorporate my special weight exercises into your weight-loss workouts. Following on from that, you'll find three sections:

1. Go-To Exercises
2. High-Intensity Workouts
3. Total Body Workouts

These are the sections where you'll find even more routines and exercises to continue with your weight loss progress with.

You'll find options for body weight and weights (using household items), so choose the options that work for you. Turn the page to learn about my special weighted routines.

Weights

If you're looking to hit the ground running, using weights in your routines will double your efforts and build muscle and definition. I moved onto using weights after 1 month of body-weight routines because I wanted to get some definition happening – and to speed up my weight loss too.

You need to make sure you're careful when using weights, as you don't want to do any damage to your body. If you've never used weights before and are worried about hurting yourself, take it slow, refer back to the form chapter (Chapter 3) and if you do feel pain, see your doctor immediately.

Always start off light and don't push yourself too hard in the first few days. If you can't complete the reps in the amount of sets stipulated, then the weight you're using is too heavy. Make sure you change to a lighter one and work your way up slowly. The reps and sets should be challenging, but not impossible.

Below you'll find a 14-day workout chart and a 30-day workout chart that you can use to lose weight. All of these routines require weights from around the home, so are NOT ideal for beginners.

Some suggested options for your weights:

- 2 x 2 or 3-litre milk bottles
- 5-10 lbs bag of potatoes (2-4 kg)
- 2-3 heavy, hardcover books
- 2 x cans of soup or any liquid-in-a-can
- 2 x coffee considers (fill with sand for heavier weights)
- 2 x water bottles (1-litre or more)
- 2 x bulk items like rice or beans - 5-10 lbs (2-4 kg)
- Your kids!

If you want to buy weights (remember, they are NOT required to do these weighted exercises), these are some suggestions:

- Dumbbells
- Kettle bells

Some suggested weight sizes for dumbbells or kettle bells:

- 3 sets of dumbbells (weight will depend on your level)
    - Beginner: start with smaller weights – 4.4 lbs (4.2 x 2kg), 11 lbs (2 x 5kg) and 22 lbs (2 x 10kg)
    - Intermediate: start with 11 lbs (2 x 5kg), 22 lbs (2 x 10kg) and 33 lbs (2 x 15kg)

- o   Advanced: start with 44 lbs (2 x 20kg), 66 lbs (2 x 30kg) and 110 lbs (2 x 50kg)

- 2 kettle bells (weight will depend on your level)
  - o   Beginner: start with 17.5 lbs (1 x 8kg) and 26.4 lbs (1 x 12kg)
  - o   Intermediate: start with 26.4 lbs (1 x 12kg) and 35.2 lbs (1 x 16kg)
  - o   Advanced: start with 35.2 lbs (1 x 16kg) and 57.3 lbs (1 x 26kg)

It's not always about how much weight you're lifting; it's about correct form and the amount of sets you do. Keep this in mind when deciding on what weight options you choose.

I typically use coffee canisters filled with sand for my arm exercises, milk bottles and bags of potatoes for leg exercises and heavy, hardcover books for core exercises. I will not need to go heavier than these for my body shape and ideal weight.

This will be different for you, so it's important that initially you start out using only your body weight and then slowly introduce these weight options, particularly if you haven't exercised for a while.

Weighted Hacks

Hack 1 - Instead of dumbbells, you can use 1-litre, 1.5-litre and 2-litre bottles. Where possible, make sure they are just filled with water. You don't want a bottle of Coke bursting on you mid-workout. Believe me, it's not pretty!

Hack 2 - Instead of kettle bells, you can use bags of sugar, rice, flour, etc., anything that you can purchase in bulk and that weighs more than 2.2 lbs (1kg).

14-Day Workout - Kick-starting the Weight Loss

Use this if you haven't been exercising for a while and need to ease yourself back into using weights again.

14-Day Program - Weights

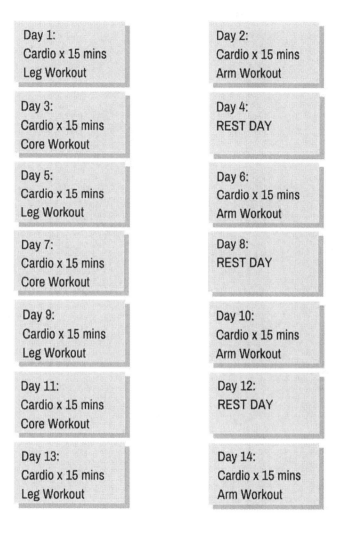

Day 1:
Cardio x 15 mins
Leg Workout

Day 2:
Cardio x 15 mins
Arm Workout

Day 3:
Cardio x 15 mins
Core Workout

Day 4:
REST DAY

Day 5:
Cardio x 15 mins
Leg Workout

Day 6:
Cardio x 15 mins
Arm Workout

Day 7:
Cardio x 15 mins
Core Workout

Day 8:
REST DAY

Day 9:
Cardio x 15 mins
Leg Workout

Day 10:
Cardio x 15 mins
Arm Workout

Day 11:
Cardio x 15 mins
Core Workout

Day 12:
REST DAY

Day 13:
Cardio x 15 mins
Leg Workout

Day 14:
Cardio x 15 mins
Arm Workout

30-Day Workout - Continuing the Weight Loss

Use this chart if you've been exercising on and off but

haven't noticed any major weight loss. Continue with this routine for a further 14 days following the initial 30 days and you'll be able to decide whether you need to make any changes.

30-Day Program - Weights		
Day 1 Cardio x 20 min Leg Workout	Day 2 Cardio x 20 min Arm Workout	Day 3 Cardio x 20 min Core Workout
Day 4 REST DAY	Day 5 Cardio x 20 min Leg Workout	Day 6 Cardio x 20 min Arm Workout
Day 7 Cardio x 20 min Core Workout	Day 8 REST DAY	Day 9 Cardio x 20 min Leg Workout
Day 10 Cardio x 20 min Arm Workout	Day 11 Cardio x 20 min core Workout	Day 12 REST DAY
Day 13 Cardio x 20 min Leg Workout	Day 14 Cardio x 20 min Arm Workout	Day 15 Cardio x 20 min Core Workout
Day 16 REST DAY	Day 17 Cardio x 20 min Leg Workout	Day 18 Cardio x 20 min Arm Workout
Day 19 Cardio x 20 min Core Workout	Day 20 REST DAY	Day 21 Cardio x 20 min Leg Workout
Day 22 Cardio x 20 min Arm Workout	Day 23 Cardio x 20 min Core Workout	Day 24 REST DAY
Day 25 Cardio x 20 min Leg Workout	Day 26 Cardio x 20 min Arm Workout	Day 27 Cardio x 20 min Core Workout
Day 28 REST DAY	Day 29 Cardio x 20 min Leg Workout	Day 30 Cardio x 20 min Arm Workout

Cardio Options:

1.   One-Room   Cardio   15-Minute   Workout   (by

backonpointe.tumblr.com) - start on the left-hand side reading downwards:

One Room Cardio

20 jumping jacks	30 jumping jacks
:30 sec high knees	:40 sec jump rope
:30 sec butt kickers	5 burpees
5 jump squats	:20 sec jog in place
10 front kicks	:15 sec run in place
:30 sec mountain climbers	:30 sec water break
:30 sec water break	20 jumping jacks
5 burpees	10 lateral jumps
20 jumping jacks	5 jump squats
:30 sec jump rope	:30 sec jump rope
5 split jump squats	5 tuck jumps
10 front kicks	:30 sec water break
:30 sec march	20 jumping jacks
:15 sec high knees	:25 sec high knees
:15 sec butt kickers	5 squats
:30 sec water break	:40 sec march (finish)

2.   20-Minute HIIT (by backonpointe.tumblr.com) - repeat twice:

20 Min HITT

1 min jumping jacks
:30 sec side lunges
:30 sec squats
1 min jog in place
:30 sec burpees
:30 sec lunges
1 min jump rope
:30 sec mountain climbers
:30 speed skaters
1 min butt kickers
:30 sec lunge kicks
:30 sec squats
1 min march in place
:30 sec side lunges
:30 sec push-ups

Leg, Arm & Core Weight Options:

1. Leg Workouts

- 10 x high knees
- 20 x deep squats
- 25 x calf raises [start with light weights, such as water bottles, increase weights each week, swapping water bottles for milk bottles or bags of potatoes] x 3 sets

Or

- 10 x butt kicks
- 20 x calf raises
- 25 x lunges each leg [start with low weights as above, increase weights each week as above] x 3 sets

2. Arm Workouts

- 10 x push-ups
- 20 x overhead tricep dips
- 25 x bicep curls [start with light weights, such as cans of soup or water bottles, increase weights each week, swapping cans of soup or water bottles for milk bottles or coffee canisters] x 3 sets

Or

- 10 x overhead tricep dips
- 20 x bicep curls
- 25 x clean and press [start with light weights as above, increase weights each week as above] x 3 sets

3. Core Workouts

- 10 sec side plank (both sides),
- 20 Russian twists

- 25 leg raises [start with light weights, such as 1-2 heavy, hard cover books or 5-10 lbs bag of rice, increase weights each week, increasing books to 2-3 or swapping a bag of rice for a bag of potatoes] x 3 sets

Or

- 10 x side bends (each side)
- 20 x leg raises
- 25 Russian twists [start with light weights as above, increase weights each week as above] x 3 sets

Refer to the fast-track page for videos on how to do these workouts.

Turn the page for some go-to exercises that you can use to kick-start your weight loss or to use when you don't have a lot of time but want to stick to your exercise habit – which you absolutely do, right?

Go-To Exercises

Use these to get you started or when you don't have enough time for a total body workout:

Key for body shapes:
Re = Rectangle
Ap = Apple
Pe = Pear
Hg = Hourglass

1. Squats [Body Shapes: Ap, Pe, Hg]
- Beginner: 20 reps [with weights use milk bottle option x 3 sets]
- Intermediate: 45 reps [with weights use sand-filled coffee canisters x 3 sets]
- Advanced: 60 reps [with weights use 5-10 lbs bag of potatoes x 3 sets]

Repeat 3 times.

Refer to the image below to see how to do this exercise with correct form.

Beginners, you might find it helpful to use a chair to help you with this exercise. Pretend you're going to sit on the chair and hover just above it when you feel the back of your thighs grazing the chair (think hamstrings).

When doing this exercise, you want to keep your weight in your heels, pushing down through your heels when you squat and then also pushing up through your heels when you stand. Do not over-extend your knee or lock it in place on your way up. Instead, keep knees soft and don't straighten them on your way up. This will keep your leg muscles engaged at all times.

How-to:

1. Start with your feet shoulder-width apart, with your toes slightly pointing outwards.
2. Pull your belly into your back, so that you've got proper support.
3. Lower your bum to the floor, stopping about halfway down. This action should be like you were about to sit in a chair, so stick your bum out but keep your chest and head level.

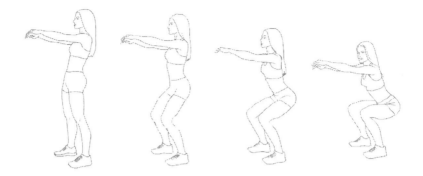

2. Mountain Climbers [Body Shapes: Ap, Pe, Hg]

- Beginner: 10 reps
- Intermediate: 35 reps
- Advanced: 50 reps

Refer to the image below to see how to do this exercise with the correct form.

The key to doing this exercise right is to keep your upper body tight, tummy muscles pulled in, and pushing all your weight through your legs.

How-to:

1. Start with your feet slightly shoulder-width apart, with toes slightly pointing outwards.

2. Lower your body straight down, keeping all the weight in the back of your heels.
3. Place your hands on the ground in front of you and pulling your tummy into your back, kick your feet backwards, landing on your toes.
4. Pull one leg in towards your waist, keep the other leg out straight.
5. Pretend you're walking up a mountain, jump-changing between each stride as you change legs.

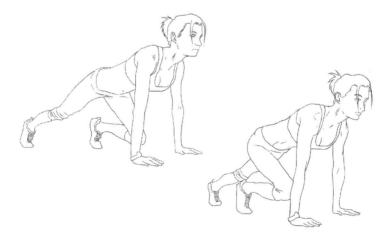

3. Jumping Jacks [Body Shapes: All]
- Beginner: 30 seconds
- Intermediate: 60 seconds
- Advanced: 120 seconds

Repeat 2 times.

Refer to the image below to see how to do this exercise with the correct form.

The key to doing this exercise properly is making sure that your hands clap above your head and that your feet are slightly pointed outwards. Do the movement as fast as you can in the time you've chosen, depending on your level.

You can add weights to this exercise by adding sand or pebbles to a pair of old socks and holding on to them or tying them to a belt; the more socks you hold, the harder it will be.

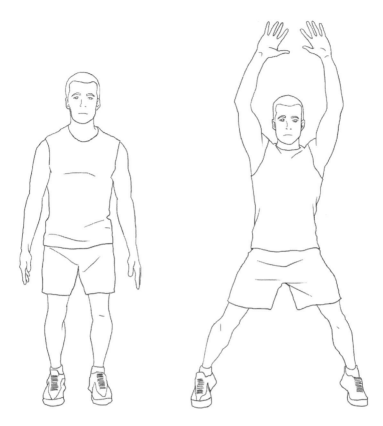

4. Plank [Body Shapes: All]
- Beginner: 20 seconds using 1 heavy book
- Intermediate: 45 seconds using 2 heavy books
- Advanced: 60 seconds using 5-10 lb bag of rice

Refer to the image below to see how to do this exercise with the correct form.

The Plank is a great workout for your core. If you can do this every day, either as part of your exercise routine or just when you're watching TV, you'll start to see a difference in 30 days.

How-to:

1. Lay down on your tummy.
2. Prop yourself up on your elbows, shoulders tight and arms strong.
3. Place the books or bag of rice on your lower back, just below your waist. Make sure it's balanced well.
4. Pull your tummy into your back and lift your body up, resting on your toes.
5. Keep your back flat, balance the books or bag of rice and hold this stance for your chosen amount of time.

You can increase the difficulty of this exercise by propping yourself up on your hands rather than your elbows. Don't increase your weight too much, as you'll damage your back.

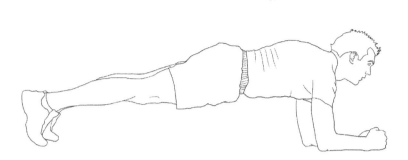

5. Push-Ups [Body Shapes: All]

- Beginner: 10 reps
- Intermediate: 40 reps
- Advanced: 60 reps

Repeat 2 times.

As a beginner, you should start on your knees; as an intermediate, on your knees but with your torso elongated; and advanced should be a full push-up.

Refer to the image below to see how to do this exercise with the correct form.

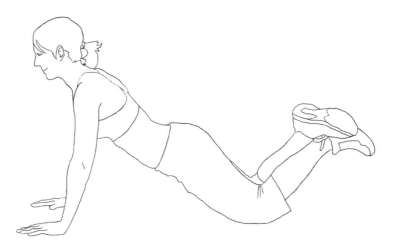

Refer to the fast-track page (http://lisecartwright.com/ ngn-fast-track-page/) for videos on how to do these exercises.

Next, we're going to focus on some actual workouts, starting with high-intensity ones so you can kick-start your weight loss the right way using more weight options.

HITT Workouts

High Intensity Training Workouts

The workouts listed below are some of my favourite weight-loss workouts and the best part is, as with every routine in this book, they can be done in 30 minutes or less! There are options for body-weight and weighted routines, so pick the ones that you want to focus on.

Key for body shapes:

Re = Rectangle

Ap = Apple

Pe = Pear

Hg = Hourglass

Refer to the fast-track page for more information on how to do these workouts.

Workout 1 – All-Over Cardio [Body Shapes: All]

This workout will get the heart pumping and should take you approximately 15-20 minutes, once you've mastered the moves. This is the perfect workout for a beginner. If you're intermediate or advanced, you can repeat this 2-3 times for an extra cardio workout.

If Using Weights:

Beginner = Water Bottles | Intermediate = Milk Bottles |

Advanced = Bag of Potatoes or Coffee Canisters

Warmup:

    20 jumping jacks

    :30 sec high knees

    :30 sec butt kickers

    5 jump squats

:15 second water break

Workout:

    :40 sec mountain climbers

    5 burpees

    30 jumping jacks

    :40 sec jump rope

    (Pro Hack: no jump rope necessary, just pretend you're actually doing the motion!)

    5 jump squats*

    :40 sec march*

    :20 sec high knees

    :20 sec butt kickers

    :30 sec water break

    40 jumping jacks

    :50 sec jump rope

    5 burpees

    :45 sec run in place

    :30 sec water break

    30 jumping jacks

    10 jump squats*

    5 burpees

:30 sec jump rope
5 squats*
:30 sec water break
20 jumping jacks
:25 sec high knees
5 squats*
5 burpees
:30 sec march*

*Weight Optional

Workout 2: HIT It [Body Shapes: Pe, Ap]

This 20-minute workout will have you sweating. This is the workout I use when I'm travelling or don't have a lot of room to move around.

If Using Weights:
Beginner = Water Bottles | Intermediate = Milk Bottles | Advanced = Bag of Potatoes or Coffee Canisters

Warmup:
20 jumping jacks
:30 sec high knees
:30 sec butt kickers
5 jump squats

Workout:
:30 sec side lunges*
:60 sec jumping jacks

:30 sec squats*
:60 sec jog in place
:30 sec burpees
:60 sec jump rope
:30 sec lunges*
:60 sec butt kickers
:30 sec mountain climbers
:60 sec march in place*
:30 sec speed skaters
:60 sec jumping jacks
:30 sec side lunges*
:30 sec push ups
:30 sec water break

Repeat 2 times.

*Weight Optional

Workout 3: HIT Legs [Body Shapes: Pe, Ap]

If you're looking for a workout that focuses a bit more on your legs and butt, this is the workout for you.

If Using Weights:
Beginner = Water Bottles | Intermediate = Milk Bottles | Advanced = Bag of Potatoes or Coffee Canisters

Warmup:
20 jumping jacks
:30 sec high knees

:30 sec butt kickers
5 jump squats

Workout:
:60 sec jump rope
2 min walking lunges*
:60 sec jump rope
2 min push-ups
:60 sec jump rope
2 min deep squats*
:60 sec jump rope
2 min crunches*

:30 second water break (do at the end of each round)

Repeat 2-3 times.

*Weight Optional

Workout 4: Hardcore Cardio [Body Shapes: All]

If you're ready to step up your workout, then this is the routine you should try. You'll be sweating profusely at the end of this routine and if you're not, then you are definitely not doing it right!

If Using Weights:
Beginner = Water Bottles | Intermediate = Milk Bottles | Advanced = Bag of Potatoes or Coffee Canisters

Warmup:
    20 jumping jacks
    :30 sec high knees
    :30 sec butt kickers
    5 jump squats

Workout:
    :50 sec jumping jacks
    :15 sec rest/water
    :50 sec jumping jacks
    :15 sec rest
    :50 sec butt kicks
    :15 sec rest
    :50 sec butt kicks
    :15 sec rest/water
    :50 sec plie squats*
    :15 sec rest
    :50 sec plie squats*
    :15 sec rest
    :50 sec punches
    :15 sec rest/water
    :50 sec punches
    :15 sec rest
    :50 sec reverse crunches*
    :15 sec rest
    :50 sec reverse crunches*
    :15 sec rest/water
    :50 sec jumping jacks

*Weight Optional

Workout 5: Core Workout [Body Shapes: Pe, Ap, Hg]

Is your tummy your problem area? This workout targets your core, building muscle and burning fat in less than 30 minutes.

If Using Weights:
Beginner = Water Bottles | Intermediate = Milk Bottles | Advanced = Bag of Potatoes or Coffee Canisters

Warmup:
>   20 jumping jacks
>   :30 sec high knees
>   :30 sec butt kickers
>   5 jump squats

Workout:
>   :30 sec spiderman plank crunch
>   :10 sec rest
>   :30 sec squat jump*
>   :10 sec rest
>   :30 sec side plank crunch (right)
>   :10 sec rest
>   :30 sec side plank crunch (left)
>   :10 sec rest
>   :30 sec mountain climbers
>   :10 sec rest
>   :30 sec down dog to plank
>   :10 sec rest

:30 sec side to side hop*

:10 sec rest

:30 sec wood chop (right)

:10 sec rest

:30 sec wood chop (left)

:10 sec rest

:30 sec jog in place*

:60 second rest in between each full set

Repeat 2 times.

*Weight Optional

Next, let's look at some total body workouts. You won't see any body shape indicators here because these workouts are for everyone! Turn the page to learn more.

Total Body Workouts

The routines below consist of all-over workouts that can be done in 30 minutes or less. No matter what your body shape, these workouts will work every part of your body. I'd recommend doing these workouts if you're happy with the body you have but want to develop your exercise habit. Once you've reached a weight-loss plateau, these workouts will also help.

Change your workouts every 2-3 months for maximum weight loss and to stave off boredom!

It's important to note that doing the same exercises causes muscle memory, which can prevent further improvement, so you should be aiming to change your workouts regularly.

Refer to the fast-track page for more information on how to do these workouts.

Total Body Workout 1

This routine is a great cardio workout. No weights needed, just use your body weight as resistance.

Warmup:
    20 jumping jacks
    :30 sec high knees
    :30 sec butt kickers

5 jump squats

Workout: Do each move for 60 seconds each
Jumping Jacks
Squats (beginners, Wall Sit)
Push-Ups
Bicycle Crunches
Burpees
Alternating Lunges (keep it even though)
Tricep Dips
Front Kicks
Plies with Upright Row
Bicycle Crunches
Shoulder Press (Squat Press for intermediate/advanced)
High Knees
Squats (Squat Jumps for intermediate/advanced)
Bicep Curls
Plank (Plank Punches for intermediate/advanced)

Rest for 40 seconds. Repeat 2-3 times if you want a longer workout.

Total Body Workout 2
This workout can be done with or without weights. Choose the level that best suits your needs.

If Using Weights:
Beginner = Water Bottles | Intermediate = Milk Bottles | Advanced = Bag of Potatoes or Coffee Canisters

Warmup:

    20 jumping jacks

    :30 sec high knees

    :30 sec butt kickers

    5 jump squats

Workout:

    Squats x 30*

    Seated Calf Raise x 30

    Push-ups x 30

    Tricep Dips x 30*

    Plank :30 seconds

    Walking Lunges x 30*

    Plie Squats x 30*

Have a 35 second rest then repeat again.

*Weight Optional

Total Body Workout 3

This workout is separated into each target body area, so that you can make sure you're working all the major muscle groups. Add weights for an additional challenge where indicated.

If Using Weights:

Beginner = Water Bottles | Intermediate = Milk Bottles | Advanced = Bag of Potatoes or Coffee Canisters

Warmup:
>20 jumping jacks
>:30 sec high knees
>:30 sec butt kickers
>5 jump squats

Workout:
Arms
>5 push-ups
>1 full bridge
>10 tricep dips
>10 incline push-ups
>5 burpees

:30 second water break

Legs
>10 squats*
>20 walking lunges*
>10 side lunges*
>15 standing calf raises*
>5 jump squats*

:30 second water break

Back
>20 bird-dogs
>:30 sec superman
>1 full bridge
>15 short bridges

:30 sec superman

:30 second water break

Core

:30 sec plank
15 vertical leg crunches*
20 oblique crunches
:20 sec side plank (each side)
:30 sec plank

Repeat again for a 30 minute workout.

*Weight Optional

Total Body Workout 4

This is a good cardio workout that will have you puffing after one round!

If Using Weights:

Beginner = Water Bottles | Intermediate = Milk Bottles | Advanced = Bag of Potatoes or Coffee Canisters

Warmup:

20 jumping jacks
:30 sec high knees
:30 sec butt kickers
5 jump squats

Workout:

50 jumping jacks

10 push-ups (kneeling for beginners)

:30 sec superman

10 walking lunges*

10 side lunges (each leg)*

30 Russian twists*

45 jumping jacks

:30 sec jump rope

15 side-to-side jumps

15 tricep dips

10 incline push-ups

30 vertical leg crunches*

50 bicycles

20 bird-dogs

:30 sec plank

15 short bridges

10 standing calf raises*

Rest for 45 seconds then repeat again.

*Weight Optional

Total Body Workout 5

This is the ultimate total-body workout. Do this if you are really looking to push yourself!

Warmup:

20 jumping jacks

:30 sec high knees

:30 sec butt kickers

5 jump squats

Workout:
:60 sec high knees
:60 sec jumping jacks
:60 sec running in place
:60 sec jump rope
:60 sec skipping in place

:30 second water break

Circuit 1:
20 squats
15 squat jumps
30 burpees
Repeat 3 times

:30 second water break

Circuit 2:
20 mountain climbers
15 push-ups
10 bridges
Repeat 3 times

:30 second water break

Circuit 3:
20 alternating lunges
15 plie squats

10 standing calf raises
Repeat 3 times

:30 second water break

Repeat again if you haven't reached 30 minutes. If you find that you do this in less than 20 minutes, add another set to each circuit, so you repeat them 4 times rather than 3.

In the next section, we're going to focus on maintaining your ideal weight. Maintaining your weight needs to be approached a little differently than losing weight and the routines you'll see will reflect this. You can't rest on your laurels once you get to this point, so read on to learn how to ensure you don't.

CHAPTER 5 - WEIGHT MAINTENANCE

Maintaining Your Ideal Weight

Welcome to the section on **Maintaining Weigh**t. This section is for those of you who have reached your ideal weight and are now looking to maintain your optimal body and stay fit and healthy. The routines, hacks and ideas presented throughout this section will focus on ways to keep your weight steady and consistent.

A word of warning here - it can be very easy to fall "off the wagon" and get lazy with your weight maintenance. But you've just lost all this weight, if you want to stay looking hot and feeling amazing, this is the point where you need to just stick with it. Remember, without action, nothing changes and nothing gets done. Do whatever it takes to keep exercise in your schedule and guard that 30-minute time slot because that's still all it takes to keep the weight off: 30 minutes a day, 3-4 times a week.

Knowing your body shape will also help with this section too, but it's not as necessary as when you're trying to lose the weight. Weight maintenance is all about *maintaining*, which doesn't require you to focus on any specific areas of your body. It's more about focusing on regular exercise and doing more total body workouts than anything else. Of course, if you're eating a whole bunch of junk food, weight is going to pile back on, so find that balance and take note of the "hacks" for tips on how to manage the food issue - particularly if you're a foodie like I am!

As with the last section, you will find workouts based on body weight and workouts based on using household items as weights. Choose what works best for your situation, with the main key distinction being to keep exercising in your schedule.

Once you reach your ideal weight, you're most at risk of putting weight on because mentally, you think you've done the hard work, now it's time to relax, and it's that kind of thinking that will get you into a whole lot of trouble.

The best part about weight maintenance is that a lot of it is a combination of eating the right foods and exercising. While you might not think that's so great, it does make it much easier to control and maintain your weight. I've found that if I exercise 4 times per week and eat right 5 days out of 7, I can easily maintain my weight, and this is still only working out 30 minutes on those days; just like when I was losing weight, I'm all about **minimum viable input but maximum outcomes**.

I tend to focus more on cardio workouts now, but have also introduced some weighted workouts (using my special household weight exercises) to continue to build and support my muscles. So in a typical week, my routine consists of 4 days of cardio and 2 days of weights. The 2 days of weights are combined with 2 of my cardio days. You'll get a feel for this when you look at the 30-day programs outlined below.

Like before, the routines in this section are split into body-weight routines and weighted routines, so you can choose what works best for you. The 30-day programs give you the option of either/or.

Remember, weight maintenance is all about consistency and regularity. If you don't exercise for longer than a month, for whatever reason, your best option is to go back to the weight loss section, particularly if you put weight back on during that month off, and get yourself back to your ideal weight and then come back here and STICK TO IT!

I'm giving you everything that you need to do this, but you still have to do the work. And let's be real here: how hard is it to exercise for 30 minutes a day, 4 days a week? If you're honest with yourself and me, it's not hard at all.

Top 10 Replacement Food Suggestions

While maintaining your weight, you might have stopped focusing on your diet, easing up a bit on what you eat as you've reached your ideal weight. A word of caution here - you still need to be vigilant with what you eat, although not like you were on a diet. To help, use these food replacement suggestions and aim to use them 5 out of 7 days during the week:

- Replace white rice with Quinoa. Quinoa has 150% more fibre and 100% more protein, so it's an easy option.
- Big mayo fan? You're eating a lot of sugar and saturated fat when you do. Try replacing it with mustard instead. There's no sugar or saturated fat there.
- Replace vegetable oil with coconut oil. Coconut oil has been shown to support weight loss, whereas vegetable oil is higher in bad fats. It's an easy switch.
- Do you find yourself snacking on potato chips? You're eating your calories again. Try replacing with air-popped popcorn, and not the stuff that comes in a microwave bag!
- Replace flour with coconut flour. Coconut flour has less carbs and way more fibre than regular white flour. Perfect if you're gluten intolerant too.
- While any type of lettuce is good, romaine is better. Romaine has more than 17 times the vitamin A and 4 times the vitamin K levels. It's the healthier option.
- Replace processed peanut butter with almond butter. Processed peanut butter

has high levels of bad vegetable oils and sugars; almond butter does not.

- Have you gotten used to having a sports drink after your workout? Replace it with coconut water, which has less than 1/2 the sugar and over 16 times the potassium compared to sports drinks.
- Replace milk with almond milk. Normal milk has 6 times more sugar compared to almond milk. Tastes better too.
- Replace breadcrumbs with chia seeds. They have way more fibre, more protein and less sodium than breadcrumbs.

A Word on Regularity

As I mentioned, the key to keeping any weight off is consistent, deliberate exercise and a good eating plan. You don't need to stick to any specific diet here. You know what you should be avoiding (fast food, processed foods, etc.), and you should definitely give yourself a 24-hour period of "cheating", where you can eat whatever you like. Just aim to eat right 5 days out of 7 and you'll find the weight stays off much easier.

Ready to keep that weight off and maintain that awesome body of yours? Turn the page and let's get started...

Body Weight Routines

Body-weight routines are your best option when you're travelling or don't have access to weights. Personally, when maintaining my weight, I like to use different types of weights in my routines, because I want to keep my muscles strong and toned. You can still achieve this with body-weight routines, but when you're maintaining, it's always good to add in a bit of resistance where you can, which is why I like weights. My go-to household weight options are heavy hardcover books and sand-filled coffee canisters.

As I've said throughout this book, you don't want to do any damage to yourself. Make sure you've got the right form and are following the safety best practices outlined in Chapter 3. If you feel a pinch, twinge or pain when you're performing any exercise, stop what you're doing and stretch out. If any of these symptoms continue, see your doctor. Don't mess around with any of this, either; it's not worth the potential risk.

Exercising should challenge you, but it shouldn't cause you any pain while you're working out. Be aware of how your body is coping and make the right call if you're in pain. No one needs to be a hero here – the only person who'll suffer is you.

For me, I worked my way through lots of different

routines until I found the ones that worked best for me. So you know the drill: if you're not sure, chat with your doctor. 'Nuff said.

You're here to maintain your weight, so don't start off light. You'll notice that there is no "beginner" option here because you're not a beginner when you get to the weight maintenance point.

You'll be able to nail most of these exercises anyway, so if you want to push yourself out of your comfort zone a little, opt for a mixture of intermediate and advanced workouts over your 4-day exercise period.

Below you'll find two 30-day workouts that you can use to maintain your weight. As mentioned above, these routines DO NOT require any weights, so are ideal if you're travelling or just don't like weights.

30-Day Workout - Maintaining the Weight Loss Part 1

This routine is a mixture of cardio and body-weight routines. This is a good place to start and ease you into a weight maintenance routine.

30-Day Program - Weight Maintenance 1	Day 1 HIT Workout 1 - Cardio	Day 2 REST	Day 3 Total Body Workout 1 - Cardio
	Day 4 REST DAY	Day 5 HIT Workout 2 - Circuit	Day 6 REST DAY
	Day 7 Total Body Workout 5 - Cardio	Day 8 REST DAY	Day 9 HIT Workout 1 - Cardio
	Day 10 REST DAY	Day 11 Total Body Workout 1 - Cardio	Day 12 REST DAY
	Day 13 HIT Workout 2 - Circuit	Day 14 REST DAY	Day 15 Total Body Workout 5 - Cardio
	Day 16 REST DAY	Day 17 HIT Workout 5 - Total Body Cardio	Day 18 REST DAY
	Day 19 HIT Workout 1 - Cardio	Day 20 REST DAY	Day 21 Total Body Workout 1 - Cardio
	Day 22 REST DAY	Day 23 HIT Workout 2 - Circuit	Day 24 REST DAY
	Day 25 Total Body Workout 5 - Cardio	Day 26 REST DAY	Day 27 HIT Workout 5 - Total Body Cardio
	Day 28 REST DAY	Day 29 Total Body Workout 1 - Cardio	Day 30 REST DAY

30-Day Workout - Maintaining the Weight Loss Part 2

Use this routine when you're ready to step things up. You should aim to switch to this routine about 2-3 months after your ideal weight has been reached and you're bored with Part 1 above.

30-Day Program - Weight Maintenance 2	Day 1 HIT Workout 1 - Cardio	Day 2 REST	Day 3 TB Workout 2 - Cardio & Weights*
	Day 4 REST DAY	Day 5 HIT Workout 2 - Circuit	Day 6 REST DAY
	Day 7 TB Workout 5 - Cardio	Day 8 REST DAY	Day 9 HIT Workout 5 - Total Body Cardio
	Day 10 REST DAY	Day 11 TB Workout 2 - Cardio & Weights*	Day 12 REST DAY
	Day 13 HIT Workout 1 - Cardio	Day 14 REST DAY	Day 15 TB Workout 5 - Cardio
	Day 16 REST DAY	Day 17 HIT Workout 2 - Circuit	Day 18 REST DAY
	Day 19 TB Workout 2 - Cardio & Weights*	Day 20 REST DAY	Day 21 HIT Workout 5 - Total Body Cardio
	Day 22 REST DAY	Day 23 HIT Workout 2 - Circuit	Day 24 REST DAY
	Day 25 TB Workout 5 - Cardio	Day 26 REST DAY	Day 27 HIT Workout 1 - Cardio
	Day 28 REST DAY	Day 29 HIT Workout 5 - Cardio	Day 30 REST DAY

*Weights are optional, not required to do this workout

Refer to the HITT Workouts and Total Body (TB) Workouts later on in this chapter for your daily workout options.

Exercise Hacks

Hack 1 - If you get bored when you're exercising, it's because you're not enjoying what you're doing. If this is you, then here are a few more options to consider:

- Dance (think Zumba)
- Hula Hooping (bonus section included on this!)
- Take your exercise outdoors. I find that this changes things for me enough to keep me from getting too bored – after all, it's only 30 minutes!

Hack 2 - Still feeling bored? Then try turning your workout into a game! There is a great iOS app called Teemo (see http://vimeo.com/goteemo) that takes you on virtual adventures during your workout. If you like to run and have an Android phone, then Ingress (see https://play.google.com/store/apps/details?id=com.nianticproject.ingressis) another virtual world that you might like to check out too.

Hack 3 - Let's talk about the cheat day. Here's what you need to do. Pick a 24-hour period (I find Friday night through Saturday night works really well!). Eat whatever you want during this period that you choose not to eat during the week - things like pizza, pasta, sweets, fast food, etc, etc.

Here are some hacks to minimise the fallout from your cheat day. These are taken from Tim Ferriss's The 4-Hour Body (http://amzn.to/1uqdXbd) - if you want all the scientific research and data on why the process below works, you can read about it in his book.

1. Make the first meal of the day a proper healthy meal. Not a binge meal. Keep it normal and between 300-500 calories.
2. Drink 170 ml (6 oz.) of grapefruit juice before your second meal.
3. Before every meal on your cheat day, take the supplements A.G.G. or PAGG - www.paretonutrition.com/ (the combo works out cheaper than taking each individual supplement)
4. Either squeeze a lemon over your food, drink a lime juice squeezed into water or drink Kombucha with each meal.

These four things will reduce the impact of any crappy foods you eat.

If you want to speed up the gastric emptying of all this crap, follow these tips:

1. Drink 100-200mg caffeine at the most crap-laden meal/s or
2. Drink 400 ml - nearly 2 cups (16 oz.) of cooled Yerba Mate tea

Lastly, you should aim to do brief exercises on this day. Definitely don't do a massive cardio workout! Do this instead:

1. 1-2 minutes of air squats + wall tricep extensions + chest pulls immediately prior to your main course
2. 1-2 minutes of exercises (see above options) 1.5 hours following each binge meal (use your smartphone alarm to monitor this)

Do 30-50 reps of each exercise. [Source - www. 4hourlife.com]

In the next section, we're going to look at household item-weighted exercises to help you build muscle and definition. A combination of both cardio and weights is the ideal maintenance program, so make sure you are getting in both, whether you use weights or not.

Read on to learn how to maintain your weight by changing body-weight routines to weighted routines (no dumbbells or kettle bells required!).

Weights

I love weight routines for maintaining weight loss. Now, like I've already mentioned, this doesn't mean you have to run out and buy a whole bunch of equipment – no sirree, if you're like me and would rather spend your dollars on other things, refer to Chapter 4 for the full list of household items you can use as weights.

Although I did cave eventually and buy some kettle bells, because I love kettle bell workouts for maintaining weight, it's not necessary. I used the household items (and still use coffee canisters and milk bottles) for a good 6 months before I got the kettle bells, so do what works best for you and your situation.

As I've said before, be careful when using any type of weight. I don't need to preach anymore here, do I? If it hurts, see a doctor. Use correct form and listen to your body.

All of the routines included here require some form of weight, so these are NOT ideal if you're travelling, unless you've got access to multiple bottles of milk, water or bags of potatoes! Bear this in mind when you're deciding what you want to focus on.

If you need the full list of household weight options, refer to Chapter 4 – Weight Loss/Weights.

Weighted Hacks

Hack 1 – Looking to replace dumbbells? Use 1-litre, 1.5-litre and 2-litre bottles. Where possible, make sure they are filled only with water; you don't want a bottle of coke bursting on you mid-workout - believe me it's not pretty!

Hack 2 – Don't have kettle bells? You can use bulk bags of sugar, rice, flour,etc., anything that you can purchase in bulk and weighs more than 2.2 lbs (1kg).

30-Day Workout - Maintaining the Weight Loss Using Free Weights

Use this program to transition from body-weight routines into using free (household items) weights. If you're travelling but staying in one place for longer than a couple of weeks, consider the household items listed in Chapter 4, as these will work in this type of situation.

30-Day Program - Weight Maintenance 3

Day 1 HIT Workout 1 - Cardio	Day 2 REST	Day 3 TB Workout 2 - Cardio & Weights*
Day 4 REST DAY	Day 5 HIT Workout 4 - with Dumbbells	Day 6 REST DAY
Day 7 TB Workout 5 - Cardio	Day 8 REST DAY	Day 9 HIT Workout 4 - with Dumbbells
Day 10 REST DAY	Day 11 TB Workout 2 - Cardio & Weights*	Day 12 REST DAY
Day 13 HIT Workout 1 - Cardio	Day 14 REST DAY	Day 15 HIT Workout 4 - with Dumbbels
Day 16 REST DAY	Day 17 HIT Workout 2 - Circuit	Day 18 REST DAY
Day 19 TB Workout 2 - Cardio & Weights*	Day 20 REST DAY	Day 21 HIT Workout 4 - with Dumbbels
Day 22 REST DAY	Day 23 HIT Workout 2 - Circuit	Day 24 REST DAY
Day 25 TB Workout 2 - Cardio & Weights	Day 26 REST DAY	Day 27 HIT Workout 1 - Cardio
Day 28 REST DAY	Day 29 HIT Workout 4 - with Dumbbells	Day 30 REST DAY

The workout below is for those of you who, like me, LOVE kettle bell workouts!

30-Day Workout - Maintaining the Weight Loss Using Kettle Bells

Kettle bell workouts are slightly different to free-weight workouts in terms of how you perform a move, although you can replace a kettle bell in some moves with a heavy book or bag of potatoes. So if you're keen to try this out, you should commit to purchasing at least 1 kettle bell.

I personally only use 3 weights – a 17.6 lb (8kg), 35.2 lb (16kg) and 44 lb (20kg), but you could get away with just 1 easily, particularly if you use a heavy book or bag of potatoes instead.

30-Day Program - Weight Maintenance 4	Day 1 HIT Workout 3 - with Kettle Bells	Day 2 REST	Day 3 TB Workout 1 - Cardio
	Day 4 REST DAY	Day 5 HIT Workout 3 - with Kettle Bells	Day 6 REST DAY
	Day 7 TB Workout 5 - Cardio	Day 8 REST DAY	Day 9 HIT Workout 3 - with Kettle Bells
	Day 10 REST DAY	Day 11 TB Workout 5 - Cardio	Day 12 REST DAY
	Day 13 HIT Workout 3 - with Kettle Bells	Day 14 REST DAY	Day 15 HIT Workout 2 - Circuit
	Day 16 REST DAY	Day 17 HIT Workout 3 - with Kettle Bells	Day 18 REST DAY
	Day 19 TB Workout 1 - Cardio	Day 20 REST DAY	Day 21 HIT Workout 3 - with Kettle Bells
	Day 22 REST DAY	Day 23 TB Workout 5 - Cardio	Day 24 REST DAY
	Day 25 HIT Workout 3 - with Kettle Bells	Day 26 REST DAY	Day 27 TB Workout 1 - Cardio
	Day 28 REST DAY	Day 29 HIT Workout 3 - with Kettle Bells	Day 30 REST DAY

Refer to the HITT Workouts and Total Body (TB) Workouts later on in this chapter for your daily workout options.

Make sure you refer to the fast-track page for the workouts and Chapter 8 for how to create your own.

If you want to try something completely different, check out the bonus workout program chapter (Chapter 6) for some extra-special options.

Turn the page for some HITT and Total Body Workout exercises to help you stay on track with your weight maintenance and to spice things up. Use these exercises and routines as your starting base and then introduce other things, like the workouts in the bonus section, when you need to do something different.

HITT Workouts
High Intensity Training Workouts

These workouts are designed to increase your heart rate and make you sweat! As with the previous section, you'll find both body-weight and weighted options - choose the one that works for you.

Remember, you can refer to the fast-track page for more information on how to do these workouts.

Workout 1 - Cardio/Strength Workout [Body Shapes: All]

This is a body-weight workout. Make sure you've got a bottle of water handy, as you'll need it!

Warmup:

    20 jumping jacks
    :30 sec high knees
    :30 sec butt kickers
    5 jump squats

Workout:

    30 jumping jacks
    5 push-ups
    24 high knees
    7 burpees

10 crunches
7 squats
5 push-ups
10 crunches
5 push-ups
7 squats
30 jumping jacks
1 minute wall sit
5 push-ups
25 high knees

:30 second water break

Repeat 3 times.

Workout 2: Circuit Workout [Body Shapes: Pe, Ap, Re]

This is another body-weight workout designed to focus more on your lower body and will make your legs literally scream. Enjoy!

Warmup:
20 jumping jacks
:30 sec high knees
:30 sec butt kickers
5 jump squats

Workout:
40 jumping jacks

30 sec jump rope (remember the pro tip!)
25 squats
20 alternating lunges (each leg)
1 minute wall sit
1 minute high knees
10 mountain climbers
15 burpees
1 minute plank
50 crunches

:30 second water break

Repeat 2 times.

Workout 3: Total Body Kettle Bell Workout [Body Shapes: All]

This is a great workout if you're just starting out with kettle bells (alternative option – heavy, hardcover book or 5-10 lb bag of potatoes) and getting used to using them. Check your form while doing these exercises to make sure you're not damaging your muscles along the way.

Kettle bell weights:
Beginner = 22 lbs (10kg) | Intermediate = 33 lbs (15kg) | Advanced =
44 lbs (20kg)

Household weights:

Beginner = 1 heavy book | Intermediate = 5-lb bag of potatoes | Advanced = 10-lb bag of potatoes

Warmup (no weights):
   20 jumping jacks
   :30 sec high knees
   :30 sec butt kickers
   5 jump squats

Workout:
   10 push-ups
   10 squats
   10 high pulls
   10 sumo squats
   10 KB swings

:15 second water break

   15 push-ups
   15 squats
   15 high pulls
   15 sumo squats
   15 KB swings

:15 second water break

   20 push-ups
   20 squats
   20 high pulls
   20 sumo squats

20 KB swings

Complete 2 circuits, making sure to allow for a minute rest before the next circuit.

Workout 4: Full Body Workout [Body Shapes: All]

Remember to watch your form and keep your weight in the back of your heels at all times.

Weights:
Beginner = Water Bottles | Intermediate = Milk Bottles | Advanced = Bag of Potatoes or Coffee Canisters

Warmup (no weights):
    20 jumping jacks
    :30 sec high knees
    :30 sec butt kickers
    5 jump squats

Workout:
    10 lunges (each leg) x 3 sets
    8 bench press x 4 sets
    5 Romanian deadlifts x 3 sets
    8 seated shoulder press x 3 sets
    12 one-arm rows (each arm) x 2 sets

:30 second water break

Repeat 2 times.

Workout 5: All Over Cardio [Body Shapes: All]

This workout includes optional weight additions, so if you find body weight is not offering enough resistance, add the weight options.

If using weights:
Beginner = Water Bottles | Intermediate = Milk Bottles | Advanced = Bag of Potatoes or Coffee Canisters

Warmup:
> 20 jumping jacks
> :30 sec high knees
> :30 sec butt kickers
> 5 jump squats

:15 second water break

Workout:
> :40 sec mountain climbers
> 5 burpees
> 30 jumping jacks
> :40 sec jump rope (remember the pro tip!)
> 5 jump squats*
> :40 sec march*
> :20 sec high knees
> :20 sec butt kickers
> :30 sec water break
> 40 jumping jacks

:50 sec jump rope
5 burpees
:45 sec run in place
:30 sec water break
30 jumping jacks
10 jump squats*
5 burpees
:30 sec jump rope
5 squats*
:30 sec water break
20 jumping jacks
:25 sec high knees
5 squats*
5 burpees
:30 sec march*

*Weight Optional

Next, let's look at some total body workouts. You won't see any body shape indicators here because these workouts are for everyone! Turn the page to learn more.

Total Body Workouts

The routines below are an all-over workout that can be done in 30 minutes or less. Now that you've reached your target weight, you need to keep it more or less stable. This means aiming to keep your weight within 2-4.5 lbs (1-2 kg) of your ideal weight (either side of the scale).

If you find any of these routines getting too easy, refer to the fast-track page for all the options, or refer to the bonus section (Chapter 6) to see how you can try a few other options to change up your ongoing weight maintenance routines.

Total Body Workout 1

This routine is a great cardio workout and is one of my favourite all-over body workouts. I get a great workout with this one, so I know you'll love it too. No weights needed, just use your body weight as resistance.

Warmup:
>   20 jumping jacks
>   :30 sec high knees
>   :30 sec butt kickers
>   5 jump squats

Workout:

:60 sec jumping jacks

:60 sec side-to-side leaps

:60 sec rest

:60 sec run in place

:60 sec side lunges

:60 sec rest

:60 sec mountain climbers

:30 sec rest

:60 sec burpees

:30 sec rest

:60 sec high knee run in place

:30 sec rest

:60 sec squat jumps side to side

:60 sec rest

:30 sec jumping jacks

:15 sec rest

:30 sec squat jumps

:15 sec rest

:30 sec jumping lunges

:15 sec rest

:30 sec march

Repeat 2 times.

Total Body Workout 2

This routine can be done with or without weights. I'd recommend a weight belt (4-6 socks filled with sand and tied to a belt work well) to keep your arms free, but you can also do this with a couple of light free weights too.

If Using Weights:
Intermediate = Milk Bottles or 2 Heavy Books |
Advanced = Bag of Potatoes

Warmup:
> 20 jumping jacks
> :30 sec high knees
> :30 sec butt kickers
> 5 jump squats

Workout:
> 10 x jumping jacks
> 10 squats*
> 10 lunges (both legs)*
> 10 burpees
> :10 sec fast running in place
> :10 sec plank*
> 10 push-ups
> 10 crunches*
> 10 bicycle crunches
> 10 leg raises

Repeat 3 times.

*Weight Optional

Total Body Workout 3

This workout is specifically designed for those of you who like to use weights. Use the household item options or dumbbells, if you have them. If using dumbbells, you'll need 2 sets, 1 light and 1 heavy.

Weight Options:
Light weight = Milk Bottles | Heavy weight = Bag of Potatoes or Coffee Canisters

Dumbbells: Light weight – 11-22 lbs (5-10kg) | Heavy weight – 33-77+ lbs (15-35kg+)

Warmup (no weights):
  20 jumping jacks
  :30 sec high knees
  :30 sec butt kickers
  5 jump squats

Workout:
  15 lunges (each leg, heavy weight)
  10 bench presses (light weight)
  5 side bends (HW)
  15 front raises (LW)
  5 goblet squats (HW)
  10 deadlifts (HW)
  20 Russian twists (LW)
  10 renegade rows (LW)
  10 flys (LW)
  5 goblet squats (HW)
  10 standing calf raises (HW)

20 rows (HW)
5 tricep presses (LW)
20 glute kickbacks (LW)

:60 sec jumping jacks
:60 sec running in place
:60 sec high knees
:60 sec butt kicks
:60 sec jumping jacks

Total Body Workout 4

Another great free-weights workout that will help keep the weight off and build your muscle tone.

Weights:
Light weight = Milk Bottles | Heavy weight = Bag of Potatoes or Coffee Canisters

Warmup (no weights):
50 jumping jacks
:60 sec high knees
:60 sec butt kickers
10 jump squats

Workout:
10 x plank and rotate (alternating sides)
15 x single-leg scarecrows (each side)
15 x squat, curl and press (clean and press)

:30 second rest

> 10 x lying chest fly
> 10 x lying overhead reach
> 10 x seated Russian twist

:30 second rest

> 15 x reverse lunge and press (each side)
> 10 x plank and straight-arm kickback (alternating
sides)
> 15 x weighted squats

Repeat circuit twice.

Total Body Workout 5

This is a tough cardio workout. It'll take you 30 minutes to complete and every muscle in your body will be screaming! You've been warned...

Warmup:
> :120 sec jogging in place

Workout:
> :60 sec jumping jacks
> :60 sec inchworm push-ups
> :60 sec jump squats
> :60 sec punches in squat position

:30 second rest/water break

    :120 sec jogging in place
    :60 sec jumping jacks
    :60 sec inchworm push-ups
    :60 sec jump squats
    :60 sec punches in squat position

:30 second rest/water break

    :120 sec jogging in place
    :60 sec jumping jacks
    :60 sec standing waistline crunches (swap sides halfway)
    :60 sec regular crunches

:30 second rest/water break

    :120 sec jogging in place
    :120 sec jump rope
    :60 sec plank

How are you doing? Are you keeping on track? Is 30 minutes of exercise 4 times a week working out for you? I'd love to know, so if you'd like to indulge me and give me warm fluffies, leave your thoughts here - https://lisecnz.typeform.com/to/gfiYCd.

So, you might be thinking, this isn't a lot of programs to work with, Lise, how can I keep changing things up?

Great question! Firstly, if you haven't (and I don't know why you wouldn't have!), go and download the workouts from the fast track page. In there, you'll find all of the workouts included in this book, plus the section on how to create your own programs with a mix of exercises. And, as an added bonus, in the next section, you'll find a couple of alternative workout programs that you might not have considered as being worthy of trying.

Ready to find out what these bonus workouts are? Turn the page to find some different ways of keeping yourself in shape and looking hot and awesome!

CHAPTER 6 - BONUS WORKOUTS

Hula Hoooping

The next few pages are a guest chapter written by a friend of mine who has had some amazing results from hula hooping! Yep, I know, it's something you probably associate more with kids, but this is an actual exercise that you can have fun with and that many people around the world are having great success with.

I mix up my exercise throughout the week and typically include a hula-hooping session twice a week because it's just so much fun. I actually feel like I'm cheating a bit, because I've always thought that exercise was meant to be painful... Give it a try, you'll love it!

Enough from me. Let's hear from Missy!

Hula hooping has made a comeback in recent years as an excellent whole body workout that gets your heart pumping while working your entire core.

That's right. You no longer have to choose between sweat-inducing cardio and muscle-building body-weight exercises. But even better than that – hula hooping is a freaking blast!

You'll have so much fun hooping, you'll forget you're

exercising! And then, almost like magic, your body will transform - leaving your stomach tighter, your back stronger, and your underarms noticeably less flabby.

As your hoop skills progress, your muscles become leaner and stronger, allowing you to perform even more advanced tricks.

For this challenge, I urge you to find value in the progress you *do* see in your body, even if the scale remains the same (or even goes up). Gasp! Because as Lise has already said, muscle is heavier than fat, so initially, the scales might show no change or even an increase, but it won't be by a huge amount.

As someone who has lost over 60 pounds, I know how frustrating it can be to weigh in after a week of feeling awesome, working out, and eating healthy portions, just to see that I've gained a pound (or kilo as the case may be).

But, one of the biggest lessons I've learned is that weighing myself constantly and worrying obsessively leads to stress and a tendency for my body to "hold onto" extra weight. Remember, weight loss isn't about being a "perfect" weight, or wearing the smallest pant size. It's about feeling comfortable in your clothes, enjoying the things you love, and marvelling at the amazing things your body can do.

If you can check off all of those boxes, it doesn't matter what the scale says. [Lise - "damn straight!"]

Why Should You Hula Hoop?

Why is hooping better than any other exercise program or gimmick you've tried in the past? The answer lies in 3 simple factors that determine how easy it is to continue an exercise program.

The problem is that most people overlook these items, thinking, "this time will be different".

1. How much does it cost?

Compared to other exercise programs, hooping has a relatively low startup cost. Many hoopers learn their first tricks by watching YouTube and following along. You don't even have to take a class!

For those hoopers who want to take their skills to the next level, or prefer the community aspect of a group, hoop classes are available through many community centres and dance studios.

Of course, you can always purchase an at-home learn-to-hoop course, if you want the structure and logical sequencing of a paid class, but need the convenience of exercising on your own schedule.

With lots of options, ranging from free to several hundred dollars, there is truly something for everyone, so financial constraints will never stop you from working out. So no excuses!

2. How much time does it take?

Hula hooping is a whole body workout that engages your entire core, so it's effective whether you practice for 5 minutes or an hour. There is minimal setup (just get your hoop out), so you don't spend precious spare minutes getting everything ready only to realise you don't have any time left to actually work out.

You can hula hoop anywhere - at home, in the park, at work, even on vacation. This eliminates travel time to and from the gym and frees you up to get a workout in no matter what your schedule looks like for the day. You don't even have to change out of your work clothes!

During your next 15-minute break, spend 5 minutes inside your hoop. Giving your body a little midday pick-me-up will leave you energised and invigorated, without leaving you exhausted or sweaty.

3. Likelihood of wanting more

One of the unexpected benefits of hooping is that it

is much more than a physical workout. There are immense spiritual and emotional benefits of hula hooping that contribute to the likelihood of you wanting to continue.

Many fitness routines focus on repetitive activities that just aren't fun. The long, boring exercises become a chore, and it's easy to find reasons why you can't work out.

The trick, then, is to find an activity that you want to do because it's fun and challenging (not because of its supposed amazing contributions to your future physique).

This is why hula hooping works so well!

When you first start to learn, you are focused on an easy and tangible outcome. (For most people this is learning how to waist hoop.) When people first get the hoop to rotate on their hips for an extended amount of time, they are ecstatic! This is a feeling most people will come back for, and is what's missing from most regular workout routines.

With hooping, the thrill is more mental than physical. Each learned trick is a new stimulus - that little burst of motivation you need to remember why you work out every day.

You don't endure long gruelling workouts so that you can have a nice body. Instead, you purposely challenge yourself mentally and physically because it makes you feel good. Long lean muscles and a toned physique are just an added bonus.

Basics of Hula Hooping

There are 4things you need to remember when you first start hula hooping.

1. All hoops are not created equal.

If you've been using a cheap plastic hoop, it's time to switch!

Many people mistakenly believe that a small, light hoop is good for a beginner. However, adult-size hula hoops range in size from 38-42" in diameter (see https://www.youtube.com/watch?v=aTF55hJJ4ms) and are much heavier than a child's toy hoop.

Think about it like this: If you wear a size 7 adult tennis shoe, you wouldn't try to squeeze into a child's size 7 just because it was the same number, right?

Hoops work the same way. You might be able to make something smaller work, but it won't be easy... or comfortable.

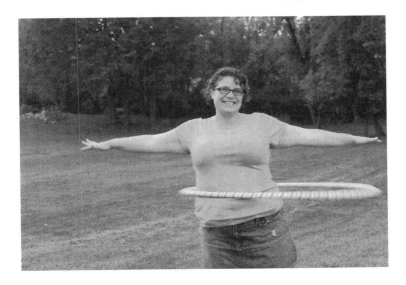

2. The hoop moves where you do.

If you want the hoop to move on your waist, you must move your waist. Think about pushing your belly button or solar plexus in and out in a pulsing motion.

This isn't as easy as it sounds!

Are you sure you're moving your waist? Try watching yourself in a mirror. It's common to see a lot of movement in the neck, shoulders and knees when a person first starts hooping.

Remember to straighten your spine, keeping your head, neck and shoulders in line with your hips and knees. Your abs, back and legs should be engaged and responsive, not rigid.

Now, wind up and push the hoop around your waist, remembering to move where you want the hoop to rotate.

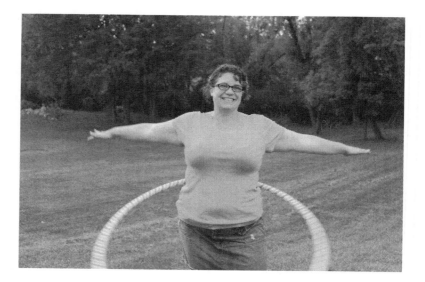

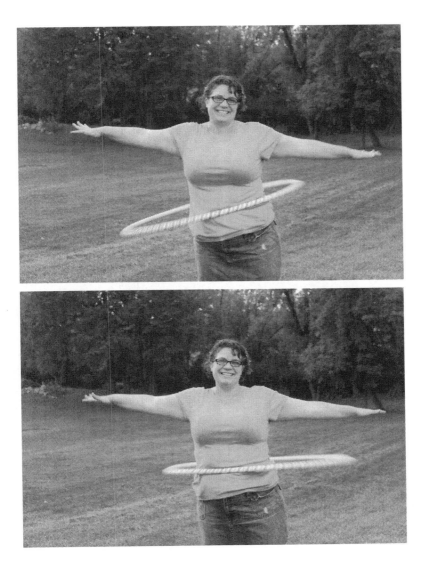

3. This is not a luau.

Although it's called "hula hooping", you don't want to "hula" with your hips (or rotate them in a circle).

Instead, push the hoop with your waist, hips or hands as it makes contact with your sides. This "pulsing" motion keeps the hoop spinning.

A strong core is required to move the hoop purposefully, without adding unnecessary movement in the shoulders and knees (which will make your hoop fall). Remember to keep your abs and back tight and engaged too.

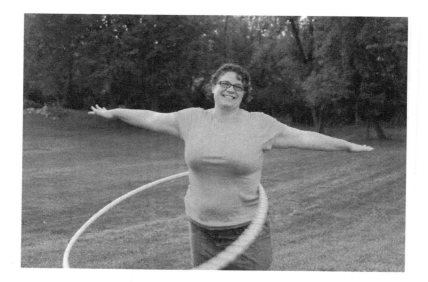

4. The hoop wants to be wooed.

If you try to force it, the hoop will fall. Remember, it's already spinning, so all you have to do is keep it going. It doesn't take a lot of movement or effort. Instead of rigour, focus on basics.

- Is your core engaged?
- Is your spine straight?
- Are you pushing where you want the hoop to rotate?

Don't worry if you don't get it right away. Just keep practicing! Hula hooping is a ton of fun, but sometimes it takes a little while to figure out a new trick or combination.

If this happens, set a limit for how long you will practice that technique (ex: 15 minutes) and then give it up for a day or two. When you come back to it later, you will be amazed that it falls right into place.

Getting Started

Although hooping is beneficial even if you only have 5 minutes to practice, hooping 20-30 minutes each day gives you a chance to practice new tricks and combinations, and leaves enough time to put it all together into a hoop flow that engages your entire body and gets your heart pumping.

This **14-day program** focuses on hula hoop basics while learning to move, dance and flow with the hoop.

14-Day Program - Hula Hooping

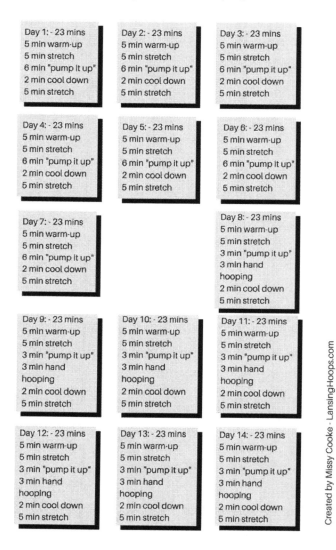

Day 1: - 23 mins
5 min warm-up
5 min stretch
6 min "pump it up"
2 min cool down
5 min stretch

Day 2: - 23 mins
5 min warm-up
5 min stretch
6 min "pump it up"
2 min cool down
5 min stretch

Day 3: - 23 mins
5 min warm-up
5 min stretch
6 min "pump it up"
2 min cool down
5 min stretch

Day 4: - 23 mins
5 min warm-up
5 min stretch
6 min "pump it up"
2 min cool down
5 min stretch

Day 5: - 23 mins
5 min warm-up
5 min stretch
6 min "pump it up"
2 min cool down
5 min stretch

Day 6: - 23 mins
5 min warm-up
5 min stretch
6 min "pump it up"
2 min cool down
5 min stretch

Day 7: - 23 mins
5 min warm-up
5 min stretch
6 min "pump it up"
2 min cool down
5 min stretch

Day 8: - 23 mins
5 min warm-up
5 min stretch
3 min "pump it up"
3 min hand hooping
2 min cool down
5 min stretch

Day 9: - 23 mins
5 min warm-up
5 min stretch
3 min "pump it up"
3 min hand hooping
2 min cool down
5 min stretch

Day 10: - 23 mins
5 min warm-up
5 min stretch
3 min "pump it up"
3 min hand hooping
2 min cool down
5 min stretch

Day 11: - 23 mins
5 min warm-up
5 min stretch
3 min "pump it up"
3 min hand hooping
2 min cool down
5 min stretch

Day 12: - 23 mins
5 min warm-up
5 min stretch
3 min "pump it up"
3 min hand hooping
2 min cool down
5 min stretch

Day 13: - 23 mins
5 min warm-up
5 min stretch
3 min "pump it up"
3 min hand hooping
2 min cool down
5 min stretch

Day 14: - 23 mins
5 min warm-up
5 min stretch
3 min "pump it up"
3 min hand hooping
2 min cool down
5 min stretch

Created by Missy Cooke - LansingHoops.com

Not sure how to do any of the above? Read on to learn all the details from Missy.

Week 1:

Day 1 - 23 Minutes

5 Minutes: Warm-Up
- Start with a slow hoop warm-up - practice any tricks you know at half pace in a "flow" or dance

5 Minutes: Stretch
- Thoroughly stretch your neck, shoulders, waist, hips, and back

6 Minutes: Pump It Up
- Begin waist hooping
- Practice spinning at slow, medium and fast paces
- Practice different foot positions (side to side, front to back)
- Practice different kinds of pulsing (side to side or back and forth)
- After 3 minutes, spin in your opposite direction

2 Minutes: Cool Down
- Slow hooping to a smooth rhythm
- Focus on breathing steadily

5 Minutes: Stretch
- Thoroughly Stretch Neck, Shoulders, Waist, Hips, and Back

Day 2 - 23 Minutes

5 Minutes: Warm-Up
- Start with a slow hoop warm-up - practice any tricks you know at half pace in a "flow" or dance

5 Minutes: Stretch

- Thoroughly stretch your neck, shoulders, waist, hips, and back

6 Minutes: Pump It Up

- Begin waist hooping at slow, medium and fast paces
- Practice different foot positions and kinds of pulsing (side to side or back and forth)
- Move your arms while you are hooping, up and down, side to side. Your arms become an extension of your hoop dance, and your workout. (Plus, this is a great way to make sure your core is really engaged.)
- After 3 minutes, spin in your opposite direction

2 Minutes: Cool Down

- Slow hooping to a smooth rhythm
- Focus on breathing steadily

5 Minutes: Stretch

- Thoroughly Stretch Neck, Shoulders, Waist, Hips, and Back

Day 3 - 23 Minutes

5 Minutes: Warm-Up

- Start with a slow hoop warm-up - practice any tricks you know at half pace in a "flow" or dance

5 Minutes: Stretch

- Thoroughly stretch your neck, shoulders, waist, hips, and back

6 Minutes: Pump It Up

- Begin waist hooping at medium or fast pace
- Move your arms while you are hooping, up and down, side to side
- Practice pivoting in the direction your hoop is flowing - first on your left foot then on your right
- After 3 minutes, spin in your opposite direction
  2 Minutes: Cool Down
- Slow hooping to a smooth rhythm
- Focus on breathing steadily
  5 Minutes: Stretch
- Thoroughly Stretch Neck, Shoulders, Waist, Hips, and Back

Day 4 - 23 Minutes

  5 Minutes: Warm-Up
- Start with a slow hoop warm-up - practice any tricks you know at half pace in a "flow" or dance
  5 Minutes: Stretch
- Thoroughly stretch your neck, shoulders, waist, hips, and back
  6 Minutes: Pump It Up
- Begin waist hoop dancing at medium or fast pace
- Practice pivoting in the direction your hoop is flowing - first on your left foot then on your right
- Practice pivoting in the opposite direction your hoop is flowing - first on your left foot, then on your right
- After 3 minutes, spin in your opposite direction
  2 Minutes: Cool Down

- Slow hooping to a smooth rhythm
- Focus on breathing steadily
  5 Minutes: Stretch
- Thoroughly Stretch Neck, Shoulders, Waist, Hips, and Back

Day 5 - 23 Minutes

5 Minutes: Warm-Up
- Start with a slow hoop warm-up - practice any tricks you know at half pace in a "flow" or dance
  5 Minutes: Stretch
- Thoroughly stretch your neck, shoulders, waist, hips, and back
  6 Minutes: Pump It Up
- Begin waist hoop dancing at medium or fast pace
- Practice pivoting in both directions and on both feet
- Practice spinning in the direction your hoop is flowing - moving both feet
- After 3 minutes, spin in your opposite direction
  2 Minutes: Cool Down
- Slow hooping to a smooth rhythm
- Focus on breathing steadily
  5 Minutes: Stretch
- Thoroughly Stretch Neck, Shoulders, Waist, Hips, and Back

Day 6 - 23 Minutes

5 Minutes: Warm-Up
- Start with a slow hoop warm-up - practice any tricks you know at half pace in a "flow" or dance
  5 Minutes: Stretch
- Thoroughly stretch your neck, shoulders, waist, hips, and back
  6 Minutes: Pump It Up
- Begin waist hoop dancing at medium or fast pace
- Practice spinning in the direction your hoop is flowing - moving both feet
- Practice spinning in the opposite direction your hoop is flowing - moving both feet
- After 3 minutes, spin in your opposite direction
  2 Minutes: Cool Down
- Slow hooping to a smooth rhythm
- Focus on breathing steadily
  5 Minutes: Stretch
- Thoroughly Stretch Neck, Shoulders, Waist, Hips, and Back

Day 7 - 23 Minutes

5 Minutes: Warm-Up
- Start with a slow hoop warm-up - practice any tricks you know at half pace in a "flow" or dance
  5 Minutes: Stretch
- Thoroughly stretch your neck, shoulders, waist, hips, and back
  6 Minutes: Pump It Up
- Begin waist hoop dancing at medium or fast pace

- Practice spinning in both directions - moving both feet
- Practice hooping on your chest or hips instead of your waist (tip: the hoop will rotate wherever you move your body)
- After 3 minutes, spin in your opposite direction
  2 Minutes: Cool Down
- Slow hooping to a smooth rhythm
- Focus on breathing steadily
  5 Minutes: Stretch
- Thoroughly Stretch Neck, Shoulders, Waist, Hips, and Back

Week 2:

Day 1:

5 Minutes: Warm-Up
- Start with a slow hoop warm-up - practice any tricks you know at half pace in a "flow" or dance
  5 Minutes: Stretch
- Thoroughly stretch your neck, shoulders, waist, hips, and back
  3 Minutes: Pump It Up
- Begin waist hoop dancing at medium pace
- Practice hooping on your chest or hips instead of your waist (tip: the hoop will rotate wherever you move your body)
  3 Minutes: Hand Hooping
- Practice inward vertical hand hooping
- After 3 minutes, spin in your opposite direction

2 Minutes: Cool Down
- Slow hooping to a smooth rhythm
- Focus on breathing steadily
  5 Minutes: Stretch
- Thoroughly Stretch Neck, Shoulders, Waist, Hips, and Back

Day 2:

5 Minutes: Warm-Up
- Start with a slow hoop warm-up - practice any tricks you know at half pace in a "flow" or dance
  5 Minutes: Stretch
- Thoroughly stretch your neck, shoulders, waist, hips, and back
  3 Minutes: Pump It Up
- Begin waist hoop dancing at medium pace
- Practice spiralling the hoop from your hips to your chest and back down again
- Continue footwork practice
  3 Minutes: Hand Hooping
- Practice outward vertical hand hooping
  2 Minutes: Cool Down
- Slow hooping to a smooth rhythm
- Focus on breathing steadily
  5 Minutes: Stretch
- Thoroughly Stretch Neck, Shoulders, Waist, Hips, and Back

Day 3:

5 Minutes: Warm-Up

- Start with a slow hoop warm-up - practice any tricks you know at half pace in a "flow" or dance

  5 Minutes: Stretch
- Thoroughly stretch your neck, shoulders, waist, hips, and back

  3 Minutes: Pump It Up
- Begin waist hoop dancing at medium pace
- Practice spiralling the hoop from your hips to your chest and back down again
- Continue footwork practice

  3 Minutes: Hand Hooping
- Practice inward and outward vertical hand hooping
- Practice "prayer hands" vertical hand hooping

  2 Minutes: Cool Down
- Slow hooping to a smooth rhythm
- Focus on breathing steadily

  5 Minutes: Stretch
- Thoroughly Stretch Neck, Shoulders, Waist, Hips, and Back

Day 4:

  5 Minutes: Warm-Up
- Start with a slow hoop warm-up - practice any tricks you know at half pace in a "flow" or dance

  5 Minutes: Stretch
- Thoroughly stretch your neck, shoulders, waist, hips, and back

  3 Minutes: Pump It Up
- Begin waist hoop dancing at medium pace

- Practice spiralling the hoop from your hips to your chest and back down again
- Continue footwork practice

3 Minutes: Hand Hooping

- Practice inward and outward vertical hand hooping
- Practice "prayer hands" vertical hand hooping
- Practice switching hands while hoop stays in motion (i.e., right-handed inward vertical hand hooping becomes left-handed outward vertical hand hooping when you switch hands without stopping the hoop)
- After 3 minutes, spin in your opposite direction

2 Minutes: Cool Down

- Slow hooping to a smooth rhythm
- Focus on breathing steadily

5 Minutes: Stretch

- Thoroughly Stretch Neck, Shoulders, Waist, Hips, and Back

Day 5:

5 Minutes: Warm-Up

- Start with a slow hoop warm-up - practice any tricks you know at half pace in a "flow" or dance

5 Minutes: Stretch

- Thoroughly stretch your neck, shoulders, waist, hips, and back

3 Minutes: Pump It Up

- Begin waist hoop dancing at medium pace
- Practice spiralling the hoop from your hips to

your chest and back down again
- Continue footwork practice
  3 Minutes: Hand Hooping
- Practice switching hands while the hoop stays in motion
- Practice turning your feet away from your spinning arm, so the hoop now spins on the side of your body
- After 3 minutes, spin in your opposite direction
  2 Minutes: Cool Down
- Slow hooping to a smooth rhythm
- Focus on breathing steadily
  5 Minutes: Stretch
- Thoroughly Stretch Neck, Shoulders, Waist, Hips, and Back

Day 6:

    5 Minutes: Warm-Up
- Start with a slow hoop warm-up - practice any tricks you know at half pace in a "flow" or dance
  5 Minutes: Stretch
- Thoroughly stretch your neck, shoulders, waist, hips, and back
  3 Minutes: Pump It Up
- Begin waist hoop dancing at medium pace
- Practice spiralling the hoop from your hips to your chest and back down again
- Continue footwork practice
  3 Minutes: Hand Hooping
- Practice inward vertical hand hooping with your

right hand, turn your feet so the hoop is on the right side of your body, turn your feet back straight so the hoop is in front, switch hands so that you're outward vertical hand hooping with the left hand, turn your feet away from the hoop so you're hooping on your left side, then turn your feet back straight

2 Minutes: Cool Down

- Slow hooping to a smooth rhythm
- Focus on breathing steadily

5 Minutes: Stretch

- Thoroughly Stretch Neck, Shoulders, Waist, Hips, and Back

Day 7:

5 Minutes: Warm-Up

- Start with a slow hoop warm-up - practice any tricks you know at half pace in a "flow" or dance

5 Minutes: Stretch

- Thoroughly stretch your neck, shoulders, waist, hips, and back

3 Minutes: Pump It Up

- Begin waist hoop dancing at medium pace
- Practice spiralling the hoop from your hips to your chest and back down again while maintaining footwork

3 Minutes: Hand Hooping

- Raise your arm above your head holding your thumb out to the side
- Spin the hoop on your hand using the same

motion you used to vertical hand hoop in front of your body

2 Minutes: Cool Down

- Slow hooping to a smooth rhythm
- Focus on breathing steadily

5 Minutes: Stretch

- Thoroughly Stretch Neck, Shoulders, Waist, Hips, and Back

Resources:

How Missy Lost 60 Pounds - http://www.sixthirtyone.com/2013/08/01/lose60pounds/
What Size Hoop Do I Need? - https://www.youtube.com/watch?v=aTF55hJJ4ms
How to Waist Hoop - http://youtu.be/HbF6UM4jUDk
Inward Vertical Hand Hooping - https://www.youtube.com/watch?v=zOS_BwZ5ruo
Outward Vertical Hand Hooping - https://www.youtube.com/watch?v=sHY_OGItZn8

Ready for more? Visit http://lansinghoops.com/nogym/ to receive two free tutorials to learn how to transition from waist hooping to hand hooping and back again.

Who is Missy?

Two years ago Missy Cooke was just another miserable corporate employee, out of shape and too exhausted to care. Tired of waiting for "the good life", she traded in the rat race and dedicated her life to helping passionate women live happy, healthy and fulfilled lives at home and in their careers. Today she owns and operates Lansing Hoops, where she teaches kids and adults how to have fun and get healthy through hoop dance. Find out more at LansingHoops.com.

You can find a printable version of this workout on the fast track page as well.

Still need something a bit more to keep you going? Looking for another workout to lift the boredom? The next bonus workout is something you're gonna love and hate at the same time - it's a real ass-kicking workout! Turn the page to learn all about it!

Full Body Tabata Workout

If you're looking for a workout to get your heart rate pumping and blast calories right out off your problem areas, then Tabata is perfect for you. Tabata is an interval based workout that is high-intensity and moves from one exercise to the next so quickly, that you'll find it difficult to keep up or get bored!

The main gist behind Tabata is for you to perform each type of exercise for a maximum intensity for 20 seconds, followed by a short 10 second rest. You keep repeating this on-off pattern until you're dying... or for a total of 8 times (whichever comes first!), making a full Tabata round in four minutes.

For this bonus workout, you'll get a 30 minute workout that will leave you panting, with sweat dripping down your face and a sense of complete satisfaction that you didn't keel over after your first 4 minute Tabata!

This workout is completely body weight focused, so no equipment needed, making it ideal for doing when you're travelling. Make sure to refer to the fast-track page to download this and all the other workouts so you can access them whenever you need to.

[Source: www.popsugar.com.au]

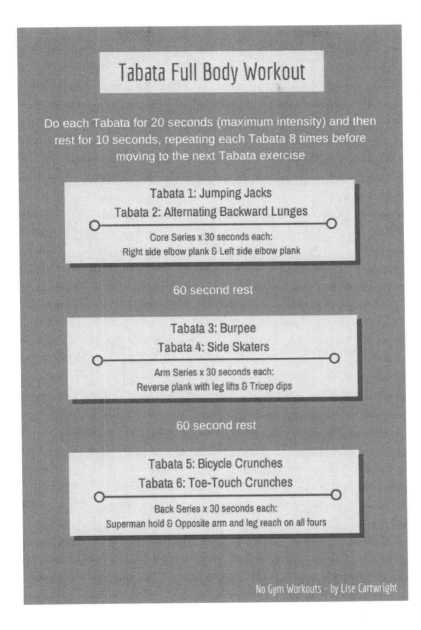

Tabata Workout:

Tabata One

Jumping jack - 20 seconds, rest for 10 seconds then repeat 8 times (10 second rest between each 'set')

Tabata Two

Alternating backward lunge (step backwards each lunch rather than forwards) - 20 seconds, rest for 10 seconds then repeat 8 times (10 second rest between each 'set')

Core series (perform each exercise for 30 seconds)
- Side elbow plank right: Roll body to right to do a side elbow plank, with feet stacked.
- Side elbow plank left: Roll to left to perform an elbow plank on left side.

:60 second rest

Tabata Three

Burpees - 20 seconds, rest for 10 seconds then repeat 8 times (10 second rest between each 'set')

Tabata Four

Side skate: Start in a small squat, jump sideways to the right landing on your right leg, then left, reverse direction by jumping to left with left leg. Keep alternating sideways jumps - do for 20 seconds, rest for 10 seconds then repeat 8 times (10 second rest between each 'set')

Arm series (perform each exercise for 30 seconds)
- Reverse plank with leg lifts: Maintain the reverse

plank and lift right leg up as high as you can without letting pelvis drop, then switch legs. Continue alternating legs.

- Triceps dips: Come to a tabletop position and bend elbows to work your triceps.

:60 second rest

Tabata Five

Bicycle crunch: Lie on your back with hands behind your head. Lift head and rotate to bring elbow to opposite knee, then switch sides. Continue alternating sides to work the abs - 20 seconds, rest for 10 seconds then repeat 8 times (10 second rest between each 'set')

Tabata Six

Toe-touch crunch: Lie on back and reach your arms and legs toward ceiling. Lift your head and shoulder off the ground and touch your toes, while lifting pelvis slightly off ground so toes move toward fingers. If your neck tires, place one hand behind your head - 20 seconds, rest for 10 seconds then repeat 8 times (10 second rest between each 'set')

Back series (perform each exercise for 30 seconds)

- Superman: Lie prone, and lift arms, legs, and head off the ground and hold the position. Prone alternating leg lift: Place hands under your forehead, lift low abs away from floor, and lift right leg up keeping knee straight and pelvis on the floor. Then switch legs and continue alternating.

- Opposite arm and leg reach on all fours: Start on hands and knees, reach the right arm forward as you reach the left leg back, keeping torso stable. Come back to all fours and switch sides.

You should be well and truly sweating after this workout. Each section (2 Tabata's + 2 30-second exercises) should take you 10 minutes to complete. At each 60 second rest, make sure you drink plenty of water.

Both of the bonus workouts included in this section are designed to remove the boredom that can develop during a 30-day exercise program. If you ever start to feel bored, choose one of the bonus workouts and alternate them with your 'normal' workouts.

In the next section, we're going to help you develop good workout habits, learn how to create your own routine, the importance of tracking and measuring, and your 14-day Challenge. Turn the page to get started.

CHAPTER 7 - HACKS

What the Pro's Know

Missed all the hacks throughout the book? You'll find them all laid out for you below, with a reference back to the section they apply to. I love hacks as much as the next person, so I know you'll enjoy these as much as I have in sharing them with you.

I've also added in some Lifestyle Hacks to help with habit development, mental breakthroughs and managing food while losing weight.

Exercise Hacks

Hack 1 - No matter what exercise you're doing, always suck your belly button into your lower back. This ensures that you're protecting your lower back at all times and helps prevent injuries developing. (Chapter 3)

Hack 1 - If you want to reduce your blood pressure and increase your deep sleep cycles, exercise in the morning, before 11am. A study conducted by Appalachian State University found that those who exercised in the morning spent up to 75% more time in reparative "deep sleep" than those who exercised later in the day. (Chapter 4 – body weight)

Hack 2 - Look at adding <u>intermittent fasting to your</u> <u>diet</u>. Studies show that you can lose 2-3 pounds (0.9-1.3 kg) per week. Start with fasting for 12 hours each day and work your way up to 16-20 hours (with 20 hours being the maximum time to fast) per day. This is a great way to burn excess body fat quickly and safely. Make sure you check this diet out properly before starting it! (Chapter 4 – body weight)

Hack 3 - Eat less than 75 grams of carbs per day while you're looking to lose weight. 75 grams is equal to 1.5 cups of rice, 2 slices of bread and 18 ounces of cola. Doing this one thing can help you to lose up to 3 pounds (1.3 kg) per week plus whatever you lose working out. (Chapter 4 – body weight)

Hack 4 - If you get bored when you're exercising, it's because you're not enjoying what you're doing. If this is you, then here are a few more options to consider:

- Dance (think Zumba)
- Hula hooping (bonus section included on this!)
- Take your exercise outdoors. I find that this changes things for me enough to keep me from getting too bored – after all, I'm only exercising for 30 minutes! (Chapter 5 – body weight)

Hack 5 - Still feeling bored? Then try turning your workout into a game! There is a great iOS app called <u>Teemo</u> that takes you on virtual adventures during your workout. If you like to run and have an Android phone, then Ingress is another virtual world that you might like to check out too. (Chapter 5 – body weight)

Hack 6 - Let's talk about the cheat day. Here's what you need to do: Pick a 24-hour period (I find Friday night through Saturday night works really well!). Eat whatever you want during this period that you choose not to eat during the week - things like pizza, pasta, sweets, fast food, etc., etc.

Here are some hacks to minimise the fallout from your cheat day. These are taken from Tim Ferriss's The 4-Hour Body, and if you want all the scientific research and data on why the process below works, you can read about it in his book.

1. Make the first meal of the day a proper healthy meal. Not a binge meal. Keep it normal and between 300-500 calories.
2. Drink 170 ml (6 oz.) of grapefruit juice before your second meal.
3. Before every meal on your cheat day, take the supplements A.G.G. or PAGG (the combo works out cheaper than taking each individual supplement)
4. Either squeeze a lemon over your food, drink a lime juice squeezed into water or drink Kombucha with each meal.

All 4 of these things will reduce the impact of any crappy foods you eat.

If you want to speed up the gastric emptying of all this crap, follow these tips:

1. Drink 100-200mg caffeine at the most crap-laden meal/s or
2. Drink 400 ml - nearly two cups (16 oz.) of cooled Yerba Mate tea

Lastly, you should aim to do brief exercises on this day. Definitely don't do a massive cardio workout! Do this instead:

1. 1-2 minutes of air squats + wall tricep extensions + chest pulls immediately prior to your main course
2. 1-2 minutes of exercises (see above options) 1.5 hours following each binge meal (use your smartphone alarm to monitor this)

Do 30-50 reps of each exercise. [Source - www. 4hourlife.com] (Chapter 4 – body weight)

Hack 7 – Looking to replace dumbbells? Use 1-litre, 1.5-litre and 2-litre bottles. Where possible, make sure they are filled only with water. You don't want a bottle of Coke bursting on you mid-workout - believe me it's not pretty! (Chapter 5 – weighted)

Hack 8 – Don't have kettle bells? You can use bulk bags of sugar, rice, flour, etc., anything that you can purchase in bulk and weighs more than 2.2 lbs (1kg). (Chapter 5 – weighted)

Lifestyle Hacks

Hack 1 - If you struggle with staying productive when you need to get stuff done, you should try using a couple of different productivity apps. I personally use Focus@Will, which I play when I need to focus and block out everything else. It times the block of time I've set aside with a timer and plays my choice of music, which is normally classical - helps me focus and keeps me on track.

Another option is the Pomodoro Technique, which a lot of people have used successfully as well. Similar to Focus@Will, the premise behind this technique is that you should have a break for every 25 minutes of focused work you do. So you set the Pomodoro timer and it will ding when you've done 25 minutes of work and time your 5-minute break. This is perfect if you struggle to stay on task and need more breaks.

Hack 2 - Email is the bane of my existence, it really is! It interrupts my day and has me hopping around from task to task if I let it. So just like Tim Ferriss recommended in his book "The 4-Hour Work Week", I now batch my emails and only look at them 3 times throughout the day.

If someone needs to reach me urgently, they can call me, text me, ping me on Twitter or a variety of other methods. But email - that is one of the slower ways to get through. I've also used Sane Later, a great plugin for your email that will save your inbox once trained! It takes 2 weeks to learn where you want your email to go and then it magically makes your inbox messages fit to one page! I love it and you will too.

Hack 3 - Learn to apply the 2-minute rule to everything that comes across your desk or even just in your everyday life. The premise behind this rule is that if a task lands on your plate, you ask yourself, can I do this in less than 2 minutes? If you can, then do it. If it will take longer, add it to your to-do list and take care of it at a later point. See also "do it now unless it takes longer than a minute" rule - http://jamesclear.com/how-to-stop-procrastinating

Hack 4 - If you're into bio-hacks, then you'll love this one. Add butter to your coffee every morning. Now you can't just use any type of butter, it needs to be organic, grass-fed butter. You should also add a tablespoon of coconut oil or MCT. This will lead to hours of hunger-free energy and focus, perfect for helping with your weight-loss or maintenance program. [Source: https://www.bulletproofexec.com/bulletproof-coffee-recipe/]

Hack 5 - Do you always take free food if it's offered to you? I do, I'm a foodie but I am also a bit of a tight ass and if I can get something like food for free, then I will. However, that is not very conducive to a healthy lifestyle. So now, I run the following question through my head (unless it's cheat day!), "If it weren't free, would I stop and buy it?" If it doesn't pass this question, then I turn it down. It hurts, but I love my body more than free food.

Hack 6 - I found the act of physically writing it down made it more real for me and created the habit faster. You can learn more about this by reading the article in full at Lifehacker.com.

Food Hacks

Hack 1 - Eggs should be on your list for healthy eating, but they can take a while to cook and can be messy. Plus, I'm not a fan of making eggs first thing in the morning; my tummy can't stomach the texture at 6am. So instead, I make omelettes in a muffin tin. Instead of using whole eggs, opt for egg whites (you can have 1-2 yolks in there). Prepare your omelette mixture like normal and then dispense into your muffin tin. Cook and serve hot or pop in the fridge and have for breakfast the next few mornings - delicious and super easy.

Hack 2 - Soup is another way to fill yourself up without adding calories into your diet. If you prefer yours creamy like I do, puree your veggies and make a soup out of them instead. Blend your veggies with a low-fat milk or broth and then heat. I personally love cauliflower and Parmesan; they taste great together.

Hack 3 - If you love brownies (and who doesn't?!) then you'll also know how much gluten is in them from the flour. Substitute black bean puree instead. Don't knock it till you've tried it. It tastes the same but with fewer calories and it's completely gluten-free!

Hack 4 - While rice is a healthier option as far as gluten-free eating is concerned, it is still a white carb and can leave you feeling pretty heavy. Swap it for Quinoa and you'll notice the difference immediately. With 100% more protein than white rice, it's a no-brainer and tastes very similar.

Hack 5 - Replace vegetable oil with coconut oil. Not only is this a healthier option, it's also a great weight-loss option, as coconut oil contains 66% medium-chain triglyceride fats.

Hack 6 - Replace all of your flour with a gluten-free option or with something like coconut flour. It has fewer carbs than normal flour and 11 x the fibre levels than normal white flour. You won't feel heavy on coconut flour.

Trying at least a couple of the hacks outlined above will ensure that you not only speed up your weight-loss process, but you'll find yourself maintaining your idea weight easier and enjoying the body you've always wanted much quicker.

Next we're going to look at kicking off your new body with a **14-day challenge**. As a bonus, you'll have two 14-day challenge options, one provided by me and one provided by my good friend Missy Cooke. If you'd love to give hula hooping a try, then you should definitely do her 14-day challenge; it will rock your world! Turn the page to learn more...

CHAPTER 8 - THE CHALLENGE

14-Day Challenge

Now that you've figured out what body shape you are and started to lose weight or are maintaining your weight, it's time to look at a few other areas to make sure that you stay on track.

Developing the Habit

I'm talking about the weight loss/maintenance habit. Without habit, you won't continue to exercise, you won't lose weight and you'll just feel crap. Your body will start to sag and you'll get slow and start feeling old. No beating around the bush here!

Don't wanna feel that way at your age? Then you need to be consistent with your exercise.

I get it, I understand, really I do. I hate exercising, even just for the 30 minutes a day that I recommend. It doesn't matter what I do, I'm just not a big fan of exercise, so it's something I have to force myself to do. What I've found that works for me is that once I've created the habit, it's part of my routine and I just do it, without thinking. Plus 30 minutes is not so hard for me to push myself to do.

This is why it's important to schedule exercise into your calendar. Set reminders on your phone, do whatever it takes to develop the habit of exercising. You want this to stick!

14-Day Challenge

If you want to kick-start your habit and your fitness, I find that using a 14-day challenge works really well. At least it did for me. It can be difficult to figure out where to start, particularly if you haven't been exercising for a while, which is why using something like a 14-day challenge is ideal. You don't have to think about it, you just have to follow it! The Action Guide provides you with the opportunity to download both 14-day challenges so you've got a printable version to take with you everywhere you go.

14-Day Challenge

Day 1: Cardio x 10 mins + Leg Workout + 5 mins Cardio	Day 2: REST DAY
Day 3: Cardio x 15 mins + Core Workout + 5 mins Cardio	Day 4: REST DAY
Day 5: Cardio x 20 mins + Butt Workout	Day 6: REST DAY
Day 7: Cardio x 20 mins + Arm Workout	Day 8: REST DAY
Day 9: Cardio x 20 mins + Core Workout	Day 10: REST DAY
Day 11: Cardio x 20 mins + Leg Workout	Day 12: REST DAY
Day 13: Cardio x 20 mins + Arm Workout	Day 14: REST DAY

Cardio Options:

1. One-Room Cardio 15-Minute Workout (by backonpointe.tumblr.com) - start on the left-hand

side reading downwards:

One Room Cardio

20 jumping jacks
:30 sec high knees
:30 sec butt kickers
5 jump squats
10 front kicks
:30 sec mountain climbers
:30 sec water break
5 burpees
20 jumping jacks
:30 sec jump rope
5 split jump squats
10 front kicks
:30 sec march
:15 sec high knees
:15 sec butt kickers
:30 sec water break

30 jumping jacks
:40 sec jump rope
5 burpees
:20 sec jog in place
:15 sec run in place
:30 sec water break
20 jumping jacks
10 lateral jumps
5 jump squats
:30 sec jump rope
5 tuck jumps
:30 sec water break
20 jumping jacks
:25 sec high knees
5 squats
:40 sec march (finish)

2. 20-Minute High Intensity Workout (by backonpointe.tumblr.com) - repeat twice:

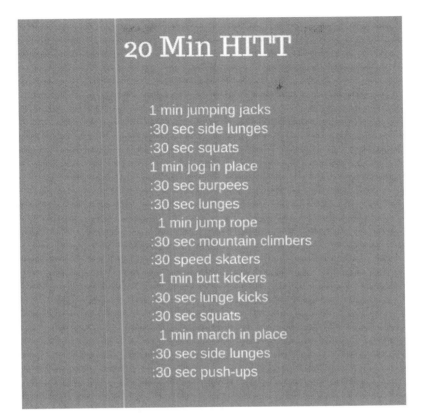

20 Min HITT

1 min jumping jacks
:30 sec side lunges
:30 sec squats
1 min jog in place
:30 sec burpees
:30 sec lunges
1 min jump rope
:30 sec mountain climbers
:30 speed skaters
1 min butt kickers
:30 sec lunge kicks
:30 sec squats
1 min march in place
:30 sec side lunges
:30 sec push-ups

Leg, Arm, Core & Butt Workout Options:

1. Leg Workouts

- 10 x high knees, 20 x deep squats & 25 x calf raises (increase by 5 reps each day) or
- 10 x butt kicks, 20 x calf raises & 25 x lunges each leg (increase by 5 reps each day)

2. Arm Workouts

- 10 x push-ups, 20 x seated dips & 25 x shoulder tap in plank (increase by 5 reps each day) or
- 10 x seated dips, 20 x wide arm push-ups & 25 x front punches each arm - alternate (increase by 5 reps each day)

3. Core Workouts

- 10 sec side plank (both sides), 20 Russian twists & 25 leg raises (increase by 5 reps each day) or
- 10 x side bends (each side), 20 x leg raises & 25 Russian twists (increase by 5 reps each day)

4. Butt Workouts

- 10 x burpees, 20 x lunges (each leg) & 25 squats (increase by 5 reps each day) or
- 10 x burpees, 20 x pile squats & 25 x walking lunges each leg (increase by 5 reps each day)

Missy Cooke's Hula Hoop 14-day Challenge:

This challenge focuses on off-body hooping, and will help tone and strengthen your arms and shoulders. Before you begin, you may want to take measurements or pictures of your body so that you can see how your body changes over these 2 weeks.

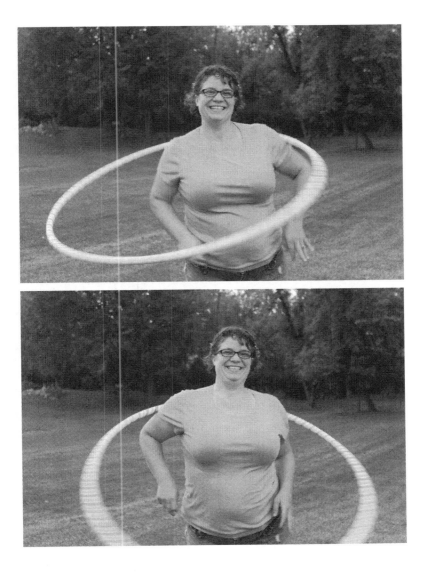

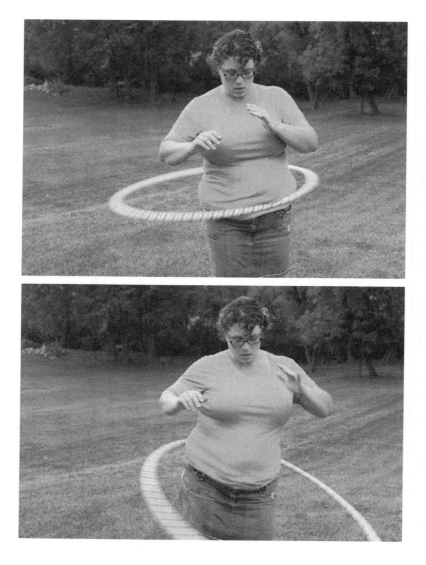

Week 1:

Day 1 - 24 Minutes

5 Minutes: Warm-Up

- Start with a slow hoop warm-up - practice any tricks you know at half pace in a "flow" or dance

  5 Minutes: Stretch

- Thoroughly stretch your neck, shoulders, waist, arms, and back

  6 Minutes: Pump It Up

- Begin inward vertical hand hooping with your right hand
- After 3 minutes, begin inward vertical hand hooping with your left hand
- Practice spinning at slow, medium, and fast paces with both hands
- Practice spinning in different positions (arms raised above you, arms lowered, arms straight)

  3 Minutes: Flow

- Practice flowing with the hoop - combine any tricks you know into a smooth hoop dance
- Focus for this flow should be on inward vertical hand hooping

  2 Minutes: Cool Down

- Relax your flow, slowing to half speed
- Focus on breathing steadily and slowing your heart rate

  3 Minutes: Stretch

- Thoroughly Stretch Neck, Shoulders, Waist, Hips, and Back

Day 2 - 24 Minutes

5 Minutes: Warm-Up

- Start with a slow hoop warm-up - practice any tricks you know at half pace in a "flow" or dance

  5 Minutes: Stretch
- Thoroughly stretch your neck, shoulders, waist, arms, and back

  6 Minutes: Pump It Up
- Begin outward vertical hand hooping with your right hand
- After 3 minutes, begin outward vertical hand hooping with your left hand
- Practice spinning at slow, medium, and fast paces with both hands
- Practice spinning in different positions (arms raised above you, arms lowered, arms straight)

  3 Minutes: Flow
- Practice flowing with the hoop - combine any tricks you know into a smooth hoop dance
- Focus for this flow should be on outward vertical hand hooping

  2 Minutes: Cool Down
- Relax your flow, slowing to half speed
- Focus on breathing steadily and slowing your heart rate

  3 Minutes: Stretch
- Thoroughly Stretch Neck, Shoulders, Waist, Hips, and Back

Day 3 - 24 Minutes

5 Minutes: Warm-Up

- Start with a slow hoop warm-up - practice any tricks you know at half pace in a "flow" or dance

  5 Minutes: Stretch
- Thoroughly stretch your neck, shoulders, waist, arms, and back

  6 Minutes: Pump It Up
- Begin inward vertical hand hooping with your right hand
- While your hoop is still moving, turn your feet to the left so that you are now hooping on the right side of your body while the hoop spins forward (forward side hooping)
- After 3 minutes, begin inward vertical hand hooping with your left hand
- While your hoop is still moving, turn your feet to the right so that you are now hooping on the right side of your body
- Practice spinning at slow, medium, and fast paces with both hands
- Practice spinning in different positions (arms raised above you, arms lowered, arms straight)

  3 Minutes: Flow
- Practice flowing with the hoop - combine any tricks you know into a smooth hoop dance
- Focus for this flow should be on forward side hooping

  2 Minutes: Cool Down
- Relax your flow, slowing to half speed
- Focus on breathing steadily and slowing your heart rate

3 Minutes: Stretch
- Thoroughly Stretch Neck, Shoulders, Waist, Hips, and Back

Day 4 - 24 Minutes

5 Minutes: Warm-Up
- Start with a slow hoop warm-up - practice any tricks you know at half pace in a "flow" or dance

5 Minutes: Stretch
- Thoroughly stretch your neck, shoulders, waist, arms, and back

6 Minutes: Pump It Up
- Begin outward vertical hand hooping with your left hand
- While your hoop is still moving, turn your feet to the right so that you are now hooping on the left side of your body while the hoop spins backward (backward side hooping)
- After 3 minutes, begin outward vertical hand hooping with your left hand
- While your hoop is still moving, turn your feet to the left so that you are now hooping on the right side of your body
- Practice spinning at slow, medium, and fast paces with both hands
- Practice spinning in different positions (arms raised above you, arms lowered, arms straight)

3 Minutes: Flow
- Practice flowing with the hoop - combine any

tricks you know into a smooth hoop dance
- Focus for this flow should be on backward side hooping

2 Minutes: Cool Down
- Relax your flow, slowing to half speed
- Focus on breathing steadily and slowing your heart rate

3 Minutes: Stretch
- Thoroughly Stretch Neck, Shoulders, Waist, Hips, and Back

Day 5 - 24 Minutes

5 Minutes: Warm-Up
- Start with a slow hoop warm-up - practice any tricks you know at half pace in a "flow" or dance

5 Minutes: Stretch
- Thoroughly stretch your neck, shoulders, waist, arms, and back

6 Minutes: Pump It Up
- Begin inward vertical hand hooping with your right hand
- Practice inserting your left hand inside the hoop so that your palms are together in "prayer hands" while the hoop continues to spin
- Pull out your right hand so that you are now outward vertical hand hooping on your left hand
- Continue to switch between your right and left hands in a counter-clockwise spin
- After 3 minutes, begin inward vertical hand

hooping with your left hand

- Practice inserting your right hand inside the hoop so that your palms are together in "prayer hands" while the hoop continues to spin
- Pull out your right hand so that you are now outward vertical hand hooping on your right hand
- Continue to switch between your left and right hands in a clockwise spin
- Practice spinning and switching at slow, medium, and fast paces with both hands
- Practice spinning and switching in different positions (arms raised above you, arms lowered, arms straight)

3 Minutes: Flow

- Practice flowing with the hoop - combine any tricks you know into a smooth hoop dance
- Focus for this flow should be on switching hands while the hoop continues to spin vertically in front of you

2 Minutes: Cool Down

- Relax your flow, slowing to half speed
- Focus on breathing steadily and slowing your heart rate

3 Minutes: Stretch

- Thoroughly Stretch Neck, Shoulders, Waist, Hips, and Back

Day 6 - 24 Minutes

5 Minutes: Warm-Up
- Start with a slow hoop warm-up - practice any tricks you know at half pace in a "flow" or dance

5 Minutes: Stretch
- Thoroughly stretch your neck, shoulders, waist, arms, and back

6 Minutes: Pump It Up
- Begin forward side hooping with your right hand
- Turn your feet to the right so that you are inward vertical hand hooping with the hoop in front of you
- Switch the hoop to your left hand so you are outward hand hooping
- Turn your feet to the right so that you are backward side hooping with your left hand
- Reverse this pattern so that you end in the position you started, forward side hooping with your right hand
- After 3 minutes begin forward side hooping with your left hand
- Turn your feet to the left so that you are inward vertical hand hooping with the hoop in front of you
- Switch the hoop to your right hand so you are outward hand hooping
- Turn your feet to the left so that you are backward side hooping with your right hand
- Reverse this pattern so that you end in the position you started, forward side hooping with your left hand

3 Minutes: Flow

- Practice flowing with the hoop - combine any tricks you know into a smooth hoop dance
- Focus for this flow should be on keeping the hoop spinning while moving your feet

2 Minutes: Cool Down

- Relax your flow, slowing to half speed
- Focus on breathing steadily and slowing your heart rate

3 Minutes: Stretch

- Thoroughly Stretch Neck, Shoulders, Waist, Hips, and Back

Day 7 - 24 Minutes

5 Minutes: Warm-Up

- Start with a slow hoop warm-up - practice any tricks you know at half pace in a "flow" or dance

5 Minutes: Stretch

- Thoroughly stretch your neck, shoulders, waist, arms, and back

6 Minutes: Pump It Up

- Practice flowing between inward and outward vertical hand hooping, and forward and backward side hooping
- Practice moving your feet - first turn in one direction, then try turning in the other
- Practice moving smoothly, while keeping the hoop rotating

3 Minutes: Flow

- Practice flowing with the hoop - combine any tricks you know into a smooth hoop dance

  2 Minutes: Cool Down
- Relax your flow, slowing to half speed
- Focus on breathing steadily and slowing your heart rate

  3 Minutes: Stretch
- Thoroughly Stretch Neck, Shoulders, Waist, Hips, and Back

Week 2:

Day 1 - 24 Minutes

5 Minutes: Warm-Up
- Start with a slow hoop warm-up - practice any tricks you know at half pace in a "flow" or dance

  5 Minutes: Stretch
- Thoroughly stretch your neck, shoulders, waist, arms, and back

  6 Minutes: Pump It Up
- Begin vertical hand hooping with either hand
- Practice flowing from vertical hand hooping to waist hooping (use the transitions you learned in the hoop chapter) and then back to hand hooping
- Make sure to practice transitioning from both hands and spinning the hoop in both directions

  3 Minutes: Flow
- Practice flowing with the hoop - combine any

tricks you know into a smooth hoop dance
- Focus for this flow should be on on-body to off-body transitions

2 Minutes: Cool Down
- Relax your flow, slowing to half speed
- Focus on breathing steadily and slowing your heart rate

3 Minutes: Stretch
- Thoroughly Stretch Neck, Shoulders, Waist, Hips, and Back

Day 2 - 24 Minutes

5 Minutes: Warm-Up
- Start with a slow hoop warm-up - practice any tricks you know at half pace in a "flow" or dance

5 Minutes: Stretch
- Thoroughly stretch your neck, shoulders, waist, arms, and back

6 Minutes: Pump It Up
- Begin side hand hooping with either hand
- Practice flowing from side hand hooping to waist hooping and then back to hand hooping (hint: remember your footwork from the hoop chapter, combine this with a transition)
- Make sure to practice both hands and spinning the hoop forward and backward

3 Minutes: Flow
- Practice flowing with the hoop - combine any tricks you know into a smooth hoop dance

- Focus for this flow should be on on-body to off-body transitions
  2 Minutes: Cool Down
- Relax your flow, slowing to half speed
- Focus on breathing steadily and slowing your heart rate
  3 Minutes: Stretch
- Thoroughly Stretch Neck, Shoulders, Waist, Hips, and Back

Day 3 - 24 Minutes

5 Minutes: Warm-Up
- Start with a slow hoop warm-up - practice any tricks you know at half pace in a "flow" or dance
  5 Minutes: Stretch
- Thoroughly stretch your neck, shoulders, waist, arms, and back
  6 Minutes: Pump It Up
- Begin waist hooping
- Practice flowing from waist hooping to vertical hand hooping and back to waist hooping (same transitions as before, just in reverse)
- Make sure to practice both hands and spinning the hoop both directions
  3 Minutes: Flow
- Practice flowing with the hoop - combine any tricks you know into a smooth hoop dance
- Focus for this flow should be on on-body to off-body transitions

2 Minutes: Cool Down
- Relax your flow, slowing to half speed
- Focus on breathing steadily and slowing your heart rate
3 Minutes: Stretch
- Thoroughly Stretch Neck, Shoulders, Waist, Hips, and Back

Day 4 - 24 Minutes (If you're not already hooping to music, turn some on today!)

5 Minutes: Warm-Up
- Start with a slow hoop warm-up - practice any tricks you know at half pace in a "flow" or dance
5 Minutes: Stretch
- Thoroughly stretch your neck, shoulders, waist, arms, and back
6 Minutes: Pump It Up
Begin hand hooping
- Practice flowing from hand to waist hooping and back again to music
- Try 4 beats for each position then switching
- Make sure to practice both hands and spinning the hoop both directions
3 Minutes: Flow
- Continue flowing with the hoop - combine any tricks you know into a smooth hoop dance
- Focus on moving with the beat of the music (count beats out loud if you have to)
2 Minutes: Cool Down

- Relax your flow, slowing to half speed
- Focus on breathing steadily and slowing your heart rate
3 Minutes: Stretch
- Thoroughly Stretch Neck, Shoulders, Waist, Hips, and Back

Day 5 - 24 Minutes (If you're not already hooping to music, turn some on today!)

5 Minutes: Warm-Up
- Start with a slow hoop warm-up - practice any tricks you know at half pace in a "flow" or dance
5 Minutes: Stretch
- Thoroughly stretch your neck, shoulders, waist, arms, and back
6 Minutes: Pump It Up
- Begin hand hooping
- Practice flowing from hand to waist hooping and back again to music
- Try 2 beats for each position and then switching
- Make sure to practice both hands and spinning the hoop both directions
3 Minutes: Flow
- Continue flowing with the hoop - combine any tricks you know into a smooth hoop dance
- Focus on moving with the beat of the music (count beats out loud if you have to)
2 Minutes: Cool Down
- Relax your flow, slowing to half speed

- Focus on breathing steadily and slowing your heart rate
3 Minutes: Stretch
- Thoroughly Stretch Neck, Shoulders, Waist, Hips, and Back

Day 6 - 24 Minutes (If you're not already hooping to music, turn some on today!)

5 Minutes: Warm-Up
- Start with a slow hoop warm-up - practice any tricks you know at half pace in a "flow" or dance
5 Minutes: Stretch
- Thoroughly stretch your neck, shoulders, waist, arms, and back
6 Minutes: Pump It Up
- Practice flowing from hand to waist hooping and back again to music
- Try different patterns to the beat (i.e. 2 beats, switch, 4 beats, switch, 2 beats, switch, 4 beats, switch)
- Make sure to practice both hands and spinning the hoop both directions
3 Minutes: Flow
- Continue flowing with the hoop - combine any tricks you know into a smooth hoop dance
- Focus on moving with the beat of the music (count beats out loud if you have to)
2 Minutes: Cool Down
- Relax your flow, slowing to half speed

- Focus on breathing steadily and slowing your heart rate
  3 Minutes: Stretch
- Thoroughly Stretch Neck, Shoulders, Waist, Hips, and Back

Day 7 - 24 Minutes (If you're not already hooping to music, turn some on today!)

5 Minutes: Warm-Up
- Start with a slow hoop warm-up - practice any tricks you know at half pace in a "flow" or dance
  5 Minutes: Stretch
- Thoroughly stretch your neck, shoulders, waist, arms, and back
  9 Minutes: Pump It Up
- Practice a full speed flow
- Combine any tricks you know into a smooth hoop dance
- Focus on moving with the beat of the music (count beats out loud if you have to)
- Remember to switch hands and spin direction while continuing to move your feet
  2 Minutes: Cool Down
- Relax your flow, slowing to half speed
- Focus on breathing steadily and slowing your heart rate
  3 Minutes: Stretch
- Thoroughly Stretch Neck, Shoulders, Waist, Hips, and Back

Congrats! You made it to the end of the 2-week hula hoop arm-strengthening challenge. How do you feel? How about your arms?

Don't forget to measure or take pics so that you can compare them to 2 weeks ago. When you're done, please leave a 5-star review letting everyone know exactly why you love this workout, and what your results were (that way other people can benefit too!).

Now that you've started, you're probably wondering what's next? Where to from here? Once you complete a 14-day challenge, follow the "what's next" area in this section.

These steps will help you figure out which exercises or routines will work best and how to fit them into your schedule, although if you've followed my advice throughout the book, you should already know how to do this, but if you're also like me, you like to have a quick go-to resource that lays it all out for you. You've got that in the workouts PDF - you're welcome.

If you're finding yourself getting bored quickly, it's time to change your routines, get outside or do something completely different. Boredom is a major exercise killer, so keep an eye on how you're feeling. If you are starting to struggle with motivation to do your exercises, then the next page will help you create your own exercises, or you could do something new, like Missy's hula-hooping program from the bonus section! Turn the page to learn how you can create your own workouts so you'll never have an excuse NOT to workout.

What's Next?

So you've completed your 14-day Challenge, you've figured out how to incorporate exercise into your schedule, and now you need to know what you should be doing next.

Don't forget to access all the resources mentioned throughout the book. You can access them by visiting the following page:

http://www.lisecartwright.com/ngn-fast-track-page

Password: 6KAZKUfVAXT4

Now that you've started, you're probably also wondering how to keep it going, how to not get bored and where to from here?

Here's the steps you should follow to make sure that you get the toned body you want, with little fuss and in less than 30 minutes a day:

1. Decide whether you're looking to **lose weight** or **maintain weight**
2. Choose how you will **track and measure** (see ideas below) your progress
3. Take a **before picture** in your underwear - DO NOT upload this to your social media accounts -

this is just for your eyes only!

4. Write down your **starting figures** using either the apps below or my Google docs spreadsheet (https://docs.google.com/spreadsheets/d/1ZgTy-kYuHK-0CNX2QiCAphTzciIPL0yoE_Odr0N6t8M/edit?usp=sharing)

5. Choose a **30-Day program** or create your own (see below)

6. **Schedule** 30 minutes into your calendar for the week ahead every Sunday night - I exercise at 10:30am 4 times per week and once on the weekends

7. Every 30-days, **review your progress** and change your program if weight loss has stalled or if you're getting bored

Creating Your Own Workouts

Creating your own workouts and exercise program is a great way to completely tailor an exercise routine to your specific needs, in particular, your body shape.

Make sure that you always include cardio and strength training in your workouts, as cardio alone won't provide your muscles with the resilience they need to support your body as you get older.

Remember, you don't need to buy weights to do weighted exercises - use items from around your home instead, kids included!

Steps to Create Your Personalised Workouts

Before you start creating your own workout, it's important to note that there is no 'one size fits all' when it comes to the steps outlined below. Along the way, you're going to have to figure out what works best for you. Remember this and you'll be fine. And if at any point this just seems too hard, choose from one of the many workouts provided to you throughout this book.

1. Decide whether you're looking to lose weight or maintain weight. This will form the basis of which direction your workouts should take
2. Shoot for full body workouts - they are the easiest and unless you love doing weighted exercises or are really experienced, it's best to stick to body weight for now
3. The areas below are what you should be working on when doing a full body workout:
    - Your quads (front of your legs)
    - Butt and hamstrings (back of your legs)
    - Chest, shoulders and triceps (push muscles)
    - Back, biceps and forearms (pull muscles)
    - Core (your abs and lower back)
4. Below are a list of exercises that target these areas. To create your own routine, choose one

exercise from each category and repeat each exercise 8-15 times, for 3-5 sets

5. Add in 10-15 minutes of cardio to round out each routine. You'll see cardio options below as well

Quad Exercises:
- Squats
- Lunges
- One legged squats
- Box jumps

Butt and Hamstring Exercises:
- Deadlifts
- Step ups
- Hip raises
- Straight leg deadlifts

Chest, Shoulders and Tricep Exercises:
- Overhead press
- Bench press
- Push-ups
- Dips

Back, Bicep and Forearm Exercises:
- Chin ups
- Pull ups
- Inverse bodyweight rows

Core Exercises:
- Plank

- Side plank
- Mountain climbers
- Burpee
- Jumping knee tucks
- Hanging leg raises

Cardio Options:
- Jumping jacks
- Jump rope
- Running (either on the spot or outside)
- High knees
- Jog in place

The art to creating a workout that you won't get bored with is to choose a different exercise for each target area, each time you workout. Make sure that you allow 48 hours recovery time between each workout so that your muscles have time to recoup and so that you don't do yourself any injury.

If you're looking to loose weight, then aim for at least 4 days per week of exercise. If you're looking to maintain, then aim for 3 days per week.

Here's a sample program to kick your own ideas off.

Weight Loss Workout:

Day 1 - Monday
Quads: 15 squats

Butt & Hamstrings: 15 hip raises
Chest, Shoulders & Triceps: 15 push-ups
Back, Biceps & Forearms: 15 bodyweight rows
Core: 30 second plank

Repeat 4 times (4 sets of each exercise).

Cardio: 10 minutes
:60 second jumping jacks
:60 second high knees
:60 second run in place
:60 second jump rope
:60 jog in place
:60 second jumping jacks
:60 second high knees
:60 second run in place
:60 second jump rope
:60 jog in place

Day 2 - Wednesday
Quads: 15 lunges
Butt & Hamstrings: 15 step ups
Chest, Shoulders & Triceps: 15 dips
Back, Biceps & Forearms: 15 pull ups
Core: 15 mountain climbers

Repeat 4 times (4 sets of each exercise).

Cardio: 10 minutes
:60 second jumping jacks

:60 second high knees
:60 second run in place
:60 second jump rope
:60 jog in place
:60 second jumping jacks
:60 second high knees
:60 second run in place
:60 second jump rope
:60 jog in place

Day 3 - Friday
Quads: 15 one-legged squats (each leg)
Butt & Hamstrings: 15 straight leg deadlift
Chest, Shoulders & Triceps: 15 bench press (or wall)
Back, Biceps & Forearms: 15 chin ups
Core: 15 burpees

Repeat 4 times (4 sets of each exercise).

Cardio: 10 minutes
:60 second jumping jacks
:60 second high knees
:60 second run in place
:60 second jump rope
:60 jog in place
:60 second jumping jacks
:60 second high knees
:60 second run in place
:60 second jump rope
:60 jog in place

Day 4 - Sunday
Quads: 15 walking lunges
Butt & Hamstrings: 15 hip raises
Chest, Shoulders & Triceps: 15 push-ups
Back, Biceps & Forearms: 15 inverse bodyweight rows
Core: 30 second side plank (each side)

Repeat 4 times (4 sets of each exercise).

Cardio: 10 minutes
:60 second jumping jacks
:60 second high knees
:60 second run in place
:60 second jump rope
:60 jog in place
:60 second jumping jacks
:60 second high knees
:60 second run in place
:60 second jump rope
:60 jog in place

Remember, you can also refer to any of the workouts throughout this book to create your own program, just make sure that you're covering the 5 areas to get a full-body workout. If you want to make them harder, add weights to the exercises. Either household items, such as those mentioned throughout Chapters 4 and 5 or you can opt to purchase dumbbells or kettle bells, but these are definitely not necessary.

Listen to your body, if you find it difficult to do any of the exercises, reduce the amount of reps, making sure to increase them by 2-3 times the next time you attempt the exercise.

Now that you've got your 14-day challenge sorted and you know how to create your own routines, you might be thinking what's left to talk about? Well guess what? There's still a bit more... The next chapter talks about a really important part of the toned body you're after - tracking and measuring. I'm sure you've heard the saying "what you don't track, you can't measure", and this is exactly true when it comes to achieving a body you're happy with. If you aren't taking note of your progress, how will you know when you've reached your goal? Exactly, you won't!

Turn the page to learn what tools and apps you can use to track all of this and don't worry, it's really simple and takes less than 2 minutes after each workout to complete.

CHAPTER 9 - TRACK AND MEASURE

Tracking Your Progress

One area that has really helped me stay focused while creating my healthy lifestyle has been the tracking and measuring side of exercising. I'm not a huge numbers person, I don't even really keep track of my Google analytics for my website, but what I have learned is that if I don't track and measure my weight loss and subsequent maintenance program, then I find it far easier to "fall off the wagon".

One of the easiest ways to track your progress is to simply jot down your measurements. I don't actually weigh myself on scales; instead I take the measurements of my arms, waist, hips, legs and chest area. This tells me how many inches I've lost, which relates to body fat. This is a far better indicator of weight-loss progress than what you see on the scales, because muscle is heavier than fat, so when you're just starting out, your fat is being turned to muscle... it can take a little longer to reflect weight loss on scales. So do yourself a favour and measure your body fat instead. It's super rewarding to see inches falling off week after week rather than checking the scales and seeing no change at all.

When it comes to measuring, the easiest way to do this is to use an app to hold all your details or you can download my Google docs spreadsheet so that you can track and measure your progress and use the chart function to make comparisons. I'm a visual person, so I need to see things laid out in this way. If this doesn't work for you, stick with the apps instead.

Here are some of the apps you can use to track and measure your progress:

1. **Simplenote App** - if you want to "write" your details down, this is a simplistic app that takes away all the fuss. I use this app to jot down what I did during my exercise session rather than taking down my measurements.

2. Tracker - **Fitness and Nutrition Tracking** - this app is great to not only track your workouts and weight/body fat, but you can also track your nutrition, which is great if you're struggling to stay on top of the food you're eating.

3. **Weight Loss Tracker** - this will purely track your weight and body fat, based on the information you provide it. It's a nice, simple app for anyone that is looking to just track their weight loss or keep an eye on their weight for maintenance purposes. iPhone and Android compatible.

4. **Fitlist - Workout & Fitness Tracker** - this is my favourite. You can enter in your own workouts and track your progress over time. This is what I'm currently using in conjunction with my

spreadsheet. iPhone and Android compatible.

I can't reiterate enough how important it is to keep track of your weight loss/maintenance progress. Tracking and measuring are important to the success of your weight loss and it will also drive your maintenance program. If you struggle with doing something like this, then definitely use one of the suggested apps, preferably Fitlist, Honestly, if I wasn't tracking my weight, I wouldn't be able to gauge my progress and I also wouldn't be able to monitor and make sure I am maintaining it.

No Gym Needed is the book I wish I'd had when I started down this path to a healthier lifestyle. There are more and more people out there who are choosing to move away from a traditional gym exercise program, choosing to do what works best for their lifestyle and their location. I have found that by sticking to just 30 minutes per day, 4 times a week, I am happy. Happy with the body I have and happy because I feel great!

I know that I spend most of my time during the day sitting, so I need to exercise to ensure the longevity of this body I'm residing in. I don't believe you need a gym to achieve the body or healthiness you're looking for, and evidently, neither do you – or you wouldn't have read this far!

I acknowledge that some people need a gym to achieve a

certain look, and kudos to them, they can spend all the time they want at the gym. Me, I'm going to continue finding and developing different ways to stay fit that fit in with my lifestyle and that I can do in under 30 minutes a day.

I know that I'm preaching to the converted here, but seriously, why does society really feel the need to make us all work out in a confined space and dress in a certain way? Beats me. It's one of those profound (I'm kidding!) questions that will never be answered. But I hope that I've been able to show you just how you can fit exercise into your day without joining the gym or owning equipment. I hope you also realise that you have no excuse not to work out because everything in this book shows you that 30 minutes is all you need.

Now, go forth and conquer... or just get your butt dressed into some workout gear and start!

Can You Help: An Urgent Plea!

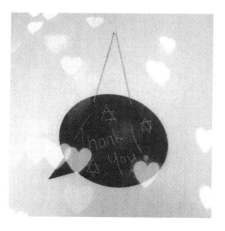

Thanks so much for downloading my book. I really appreciate your feedback and I LOVE hearing what you have to say.

So, with that in mind, I need your input to make the next version of this book even better. **Please leave a helpful REVIEW on Amazon by visiting http://bit.ly/ngnbook!** Thanks so much!!

~ Lise

Acknowledgements

There were so many people that inspired me to write this book, and there were also so many amazing people that helped refine my ideas and make this book come to life. Thank you for your support and for helping to make this book great!

Chandler Bolt, James Roper, Tyler Wagner, Carlo Cretaro, Florence Murphy, Steve Windsor, Jennifer Grainger, Karen Marston, Missy Cooke, Liz Froment, Joanne Amos, Michelle Reynolds, Stacey Clift, Alison Stokes, Ceri Wackrow, Letitia Buckle, Audrey O'Brien, Linda Knight, Jacs Blake, Cathy Whyte and the community behind BSBS!

About the Author

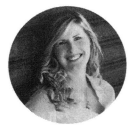 Lise is an author, blogger and freelance writer who is also a self-confessed shoe fanatic — she's obsessed. Just ask her husband!

She has been looking for the magic in life since she was first exposed to positive, happy thoughts at the tender age of one - thanks Mum and Dad!

Lise can regularly be found at local cafes, NOT drinking coffee, but the more sophisticated and magical beverage that is a *Chai Latte*.

If you're looking to connect with Lise, you can stalk her on Facebook, annoy her on Twitter or send her an email to lise@lisecartwright.com.

If you want to learn more about what she does for a day job, check out www.hustleandgroove.com.

60903952R00121

Made in the USA
Middletown, DE
05 January 2018